## DATE DUE

| | |
|---|---|
| MAY 09 | JUN 05 1998 |
| 10/21/95 | DEC 2 1 1997 |
| JAN 13 1996 | |
| JAN 14 1996 | APR - 8 1998 |
| | JUL 26 1998 |
| FEB 2 8 1998 | |
| OCT 0 9 1997 | |
| FEB 24 1998 | |
| DEC 28 1998 | |
| JAN - 3 2000 | |
| DEC 27 2000 | |
| | |
| | |

GAYLORD                    PRINTED IN U.S.A.

# The Challenge of Cognitive Therapy

*Applications to*
*Nontraditional Populations*

# APPLIED CLINICAL PSYCHOLOGY

Series Editors:
Alan S. Bellack, *Medical College of Pennsylvania at EPPI, Philadelphia, Pennsylvania,*
and Michel Hersen, *University of Pittsburgh, Pittsburgh, Pennsylvania*

A Continuation Order Plan is available for this series. A continuation order will bring delivery of each new volume immediately upon publication. Volumes are billed only upon actual shipment. For further information please contact the publisher.

# The Challenge of Cognitive Therapy

## Applications to Nontraditional Populations

Edited by

## T. MICHAEL VALLIS AND
## JANICE L. HOWES

*Dalhousie University*
*Camp Hill Medical Center*
*Halifax, Nova Scotia, Canada*

and

## PHILIP C. MILLER

*Behavioral Health Clinic*
*Toronto, Ontario, Canada*

PLENUM PRESS • NEW YORK AND LONDON

Library of Congress Cataloging-in-Publication Data

The Challenge of cognitive therapy : applications to nontraditional
  populations / edited by T. Michael Vallis and Janice L. Howes and
  Philip C. Miller.
      p.    cm. -- (Applied clinical psychology)
  Includes bibliographical references and index.
  ISBN 0-306-43629-9
   1. Cognitive therapy.   I. Vallis, T. Michael.  II. Howes, Janice
  L.   III. Miller, Philip C., 1950-   .  IV. Series.
   [DNLM: 1. Cognitive Therapy.  2. Mental Disorders--therapy.
  3. Pain--therapy.   WM 425 C437]
  RC489.C63C48  1990
  616.89'142--dc20
  DNLM/DLC
  for Library of Congress                                    90-14306
                                                                 CIP

ISBN 0-306-43629-9

© 1991 Plenum Press, New York
A Division of Plenum Publishing Corporation
233 Spring Street, New York, N.Y. 10013

Printed in the United States of America

# Contributors

Steven Fleming
  Department of Psychology, Atkinson College, York University, North York, Ontario M3J 2R7, Canada

Janice L. Howes
  Department of Psychiatry, Dalhousie University, and Department of Psychology, Camp Hill Medical Center, Halifax, Nova Scotia B3H 3G2, Canada

Philip C. Miller
  Behavioral Health Clinic, Toronto, Ontario M6A 2T3, Canada

Mark Olioff
  Department of Psychology, The Mississauga Hospital, Mississauga, Ontario L5B 1B8, Canada

Carol A. Parrott
  Private Practice, 1060 Springhill Drive, Mississauga, Ontario L5H 1M9, Canada

Paul J. Robinson
  Department of Psychology, North York General Hospital, Willowdale, Ontario M2K 1E1, Canada

Marsha M. Rothstein
  Independent Practice, Delisle Court Professional Center, 1560 Yonge Street, Suite 300, Toronto, Ontario M4T 2S9, Canada

T. Michael Vallis
  Departments of Psychology and Psychiatry, Dalhousie University, and Department of Psychology, Camp Hill Medical Center, Halifax, Nova Scotia B3H 3G2, Canada

# *Preface*

Cognitive therapy is fast becoming one of the more popular and well-respected forms of psychotherapy. In both research and clinical practice, several advantages of cognitive therapy have been identified. Cognitive therapy is structured enough to provide a therapeutic framework for clinicians, as well as a theoretical framework for clinical researchers, yet flexible enough to address an individual's problems in a highly idiosyncratic manner. Accompanying the popularity of cognitive therapy is the expansion of its application beyond the areas in which it was initially developed and validated (the "traditional" areas of depression and anxiety) to areas where validation has not yet occurred (the "nontraditional" areas). We strongly believe that such broadening of cognitive therapy should be encouraged, but that conceptual models to guide the therapist and researcher in these areas should be explicated. It is the purpose of this text to provide a conceptual framework for dealing with select, nontraditional populations.

The idea and motivation for this text develops from a cognitive therapy interest group in Toronto. All of the authors contributing to this text are involved in this group. We represent a group of cognitive therapists functioning in a variety of diverse settings, including clinical research units, general hospital settings, private or public rehabilitation centers, and private practices. Thus, the diversity of referrals for cognitive therapy within our group is great. Our collective experience in implementing cognitive therapy is that, while existing models guiding therapeutic interventions are useful, these models require modification to address the issues presented by our nontraditional patients. Both conceptual and procedural adaptations are identified. As a group, we strive to develop a general integrative conceptual approach to cognitive therapy that will guide therapists in a flexible manner. Complementing this, we attempt to articulate what is unique to the populations with which we work, and what modifications are required in implementing cognitive therapy with these populations. This text is the result of our work. In Part I, a general, integrative framework to guide cognitive therapists working with nontraditional populations is presented. In Part II, five specific nontraditional patient populations are presented, and cognitive issues specific to working with these populations are addressed.

Part I is composed of three chapters. In Chapter 1, a general overview of the theoretical and conceptual bases of cognitive therapy is presented. The purpose of this chapter is to ground the reader in existing cognitive therapy models and, as such, set the stage for the remainder of the text. In Chapter 2, conceptualization in cognitive therapy is addressed. A number of different conceptual frameworks available to the cognitive therapist are reviewed, and guidelines are presented to aid the therapist in developing the most appropriate conceptual model for a given case. The final chapter of Part I, Chapter 3, examines the therapeutic relationship in cognitive therapy. Different models of the therapeutic relationship are reviewed and guidelines are suggested for the flexible use of such models.

Part II is composed of five chapters outlining the application of cognitive therapy with specific populations. All chapters in this section are clinically based, relying heavily on case examples to illustrate the treatment approach. The treatment of personality disorders is addressed in Chapter 4. In Chapter 5, cognitive therapy with posttraumatic stress disorder is outlined. Chapter 6 consists of a treatment model for cognitive therapy with postpartum depression. The treatment of bereavement using cognitive therapy is presented in Chapter 7. Finally, a model for implementing cognitive therapy with chronic pain disorders is outlined in Chapter 8.

One limitation of our text is the lack of empirical data to validate our hypotheses. We readily acknowledge this and strongly encourage the research necessary to examine the validity of our ideas. Our view is that conceptual frameworks should precede empirical research and to this end we hope that our ideas will stimulate research. As well, we take a developmental perspective on cognitive therapy. The ideas presented in this text are initial steps, and we look forward to the refinements and modifications that our ideas might stimulate.

Many people deserve acknowledgment and thanks for their efforts and support during the completion of this text. First, we wish to express our sincere thanks and appreciation to Loretta McKenzie, who prepared all chapters. Loretta's efficiency, competence, hard work, and good humor greatly facilitated the preparation of this text. Second, we express our gratitude to Eliot Werner, executive editor, medical and social sciences, Plenum Press, for his support and encouragement of our nontraditional approach to an edited text. Finally, we wish to thank Dr. C. Bilsbury, the Department of Psychology, and the Camp Hill Medical Center, for their financial support of the preparation of this text.

T. Michael Vallis
Janice L. Howes
Philip C. Miller

# Contents

## PART I: THEORETICAL ADVANCES IN COGNITIVE THERAPY

# PART II: CLINICAL APPLICATIONS

# I

# *Theoretical Advances in Cognitive Therapy*

# 1

# Theoretical and Conceptual Bases of Cognitive Therapy

T. MICHAEL VALLIS

## INTRODUCTION

Any review of the literature on psychotherapy, even the most cursory perusal, will make reference to the "cognitive revolution" (e.g., Mahoney & Freeman, 1985). Cognitive perspectives on psychopathology and clinical treatment have been advocated for a number of years. Ellis's work on rational-emotive therapy (RET; e.g., Ellis & Greiger, 1977) and Beck's cognitive-phenomenological formulations of the emotional disorders (e.g., Beck, 1976) are examples of this early work. However, during the last decade there has been an exponential growth of interest in cognitive therapy. The number of publications on cognitive therapy continue to proliferate. There are now two journals specifically devoted to cognitive therapy: *Cognitive Therapy and Research* (established in 1977 and published by Plenum Press) and the recent *Journal of Cognitive Psychotherapy: An International Quarterly* (established in 1987 and published by Springer Publishing Corporation). Further, courses on cognitive therapy are being offered in clinical psychology graduate programs (e.g., the University of British Columbia; Dalhousie University), and are incorporated into psychiatry residency training programs (e.g., the University of Toronto; Dalhousie University). Finally, centers for cognitive therapy have been established throughout North America (e.g., the Center for Cognitive Therapy in Philadelphia; the New York Center for Cognitive Therapy; the Center for Cognitive Therapy in Newport Beach, Califor-

T. MICHAEL VALLIS • Departments of Psychology and Psychiatry, Dalhousie University, and Department of Psychology, Camp Hill Medical Center, Halifax, Nova Scotia B3H 3G2, Canada.

nia; the Cognitive and Behavior Therapies Section at the Clarke Institute of Psychiatry, Toronto). The most recent World Congress of Cognitive Therapy held in Oxford, England, in June 1989, was attended by over 800 participants. In light of these developments, it is reasonable to conclude that cognitive therapy has become a subspecialty within clinical practice and that it will continue to attract attention from both researchers and practitioners.

The purpose of this text is to outline recent developments in the application of cognitive therapy to relatively novel (for cognitive therapy) populations. Recent theoretical and conceptual developments are outlined in Part I. In Part II the clinical application of cognitive therapy to selected nontraditional populations is presented. In the present chapter, the theoretical/conceptual bases for the cognitive therapies are overviewed. Recent developments of particular importance to the disorders addressed in Part II are presented. Presentation of specific cognitive models of psychopathology (such as unipolar depression or anxiety), and evaluation of the validity of these models, is beyond the scope of this chapter (see Shaw & Segal, 1989).

As is true of sustained study of most phenomena, refinements in conceptual formulation, and differentiation of procedural applications, occur over time. This certainly is the case with cognitive therapy. For example, with respect to conceptual refinements, there has been, and still may be, confusion surrounding the issue of the causal role of cognition in depression. Early formulations of cognitive therapy stressed the role of cognition to the relative exclusion of noncognitive processes (e.g., Ellis, 1977; Kovacs & Beck, 1978). Compounding this tendency was the heavy reliance on the information-processing model, which purports cognition to be primary and affect to be secondary (see Lazarus, 1984; Zajonc, 1984). As a result, some researchers in the field have interpreted cognitive theorists as claiming that cognitions are causal phenomena (Silverman, Silverman, & Eardley 1984; Simons, Garfield, & Murphy, 1984). This has generated controversy and criticism (Coyne & Gotlib, 1983; Silverman *et al.*, 1984) and stimulated a clear articulation of cognition, not as a unitary causal factor, but as part of an interactive biopsychosocial causal model (see Beck, 1983, 1985; Riskind & Steer, 1984). Apart from conceptual refinements, procedural distinctions within cognitive therapy can be drawn between Ellis's rational-emotive therapy (e.g., Ellis & Greiger, 1977), Beck's cognitive therapy (Beck, Rush, Shaw, & Emery, 1979), Meichenbaum's stress-inoculation training (Meichenbaum, 1977), Rehm's self-control therapy (Rehm, 1981), and Guidano and Liotti's constructivist-based cognitive therapy (Guidano & Liotti, 1983), to name just a few.

Although significant differentiation has occurred in cognitive therapy, there exists a common set of assumptions which, for the most part, cut across technical or theoretical variations, and which continue to define the cognitive approach.

## Assumptions Common to All Cognitive Therapies

All approaches to cognitive therapy are based on the principles of phenomenology, collaboration, activity, empiricism, and generalization. However, it must be emphasized that cognitive therapy, as a system of psychotherapy, places heavy emphasis on the therapeutic relationship and makes full use of the "nonspecific" factors that have been shown to be potent therapeutic ingredients (see Beck *et al.*, 1979; Frank, 1985; Chapter 3, this volume).

Perhaps the most distinctive aspect of cognitive therapy is that it involves a *phenomenological approach* to psychopathology and clinical change (Beck *et al.*, 1979; Guidano & Liotti, 1983; Mahoney, 1985, 1988; Rush & Giles, 1982). Regardless of the therapist's theoretical notions or biases, the idiosyncratic subjective experience of the patient is the basis of the therapeutic exchange. It is the world, whether it be self-oriented, other-oriented, event-oriented, or some combination, *through the patient's eyes*, that is essential in cognitive therapy. Thus, all forms of cognitive therapy rely heavily on patients' self-reports of their experience, although the focus on specific aspects of their experience (e.g., cognitive content, cognitive process, or cognitive structure) varies among therapists and conceptual models.

In working from a phenomenological perspective, the therapist's task is to understand how the patient construes his/her world and how this construal impacts on emotional distress and behavioral dysfunction. Once identified, therapists attempt to facilitate behavioral, cognitive, and emotional events (in or out of session) that will stimulate change to this construal process. Although phenomenology underlies all forms of cognitive therapy, the different "schools" vary in the extent to which the idiosyncratic nature of the individual's perception is stressed. In some forms of cognitive therapy, such as RET or self-instructional training, therapists operate from a fairly standard list of beliefs (see Ellis, 1977, pp. 8-20), or from a structured approach to intervention techniques. For example, in self-instructional training, standard lists of self-instructions are often employed (e.g., "Take things one step at a time," "Focus on what you have to do next"; Meichenbaum, 1977). In other forms of cognitive therapy the therapist's approach to exploring the patient's experience, and encouraging cognitive reappraisal, is highly idiosyncratic. This is true for Beck's cognitive therapy (Beck *et al.*, 1979), Guidano and Liotti's (1983) constructivist model of cognitive therapy, and Safran's cognitive-interpersonal model of cognitive therapy (Safran & Segal, 1990).

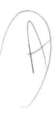

A second assumption common to all of the cognitive therapies is that the nature of the relationship between the patient and therapist is one of *collaboration* (Beck *et al.*, 1979). This follows from the emphasis on phenomenology. The patient and the therapist work together in a negotiated fashion. Again, while there is some variability in the extent to which this is followed, it can nonetheless be stated as a principle common to all forms of cognitive therapy. Collaboration is one area where neophyte therapists often have difficulty. For instance, in the National Institute of Mental Health's Treatment of Depression Collaborative Research Program (TDCRP, Elkin, Parloff, Hadley, & Autry, 1985), a common problem in the early stages of training in cognitive therapy was that therapists focused on technique to the exclusion of collaboration (Shaw, 1984). In cognitive therapy therapists often explicitly present their therapeutic approach as "it's you and me against the depression (anxiety, pain, etc.)" rather than "it's me treating you" (see Beck *et al.*, 1979).

It follows from the collaborative relationship that cognitive therapy is an *active* treatment approach. Both the patient and therapist have a definite role in selecting therapeutic targets and negotiating how such targets are to be approached. This is a relatively unique aspect of cognitive therapy, particularly in the context of noncognitive therapy approaches, where therapist activity might be seen as a negative factor. For instance, Vallis, Shaw, and McCabe (1988), in a study comparing ratings of therapist competency in cognitive therapy (see Dobson, Shaw, & Vallis, 1985; Vallis, Shaw, & Dobson, 1986) to general nonspecific therapist skill ratings, reported that greater competency in cognitive therapy was positively related to greater therapist "errors" in communication on the Matarazzo Checklist of Therapist Behaviors (MCTB; Matarazzo, Philips, Wein, & Saslow, 1965). This relationship was mediated by higher frequencies of brief-answer (Yes/No) questions and interruptions by the more competent cognitive therapists. In cognitive therapy brief-answer questions and interruptions are not regarded as errors, but are regarded as part of the active collaboration between the patient and therapist. Clearly, what is competent within one system of psychotherapy may not be judged as competent within another.

A fourth working assumption of all forms of cognitive therapy is that therapy involves an *empirical* focus. The patient's idiosyncratic construal processes, be they automatic thoughts or negative self-referent schemata (Hollon & Kriss, 1984), are subjected to close scrutiny. This scrutiny may take the form of actual data gathering (Beck *et al.*, 1979) or involve the process of decentering and reevaluation of core dysfunctional beliefs (Guidano & Liotti, 1983).

Finally, cognitive therapy approaches are characterized by prescribed activities designed to facilitate the *generalization* of in-session therapeutic change. These activities are the "homework" of cognitive therapy. The cognitive therapies differ in the extent to which such generalization activities are explicitly determined, monitored, and evaluated. However, it is generally true that the cognitive therapies are not focused selectively and entirely on the patient-therapist in-session interaction. Much therapeutic attention is devoted to patient functioning outside of the therapy context, and there are several studies which suggest that compliance with homework assignments is related to better outcome (Neimeyer, Twentyman, & Prezant, 1985; Persons, Burns, & Perloff, 1988; Primakoff, Epstein, & Covi, 1989).

## HISTORICAL DEVELOPMENT AND EVOLUTION OF THE COGNITIVE THERAPIES

It should be clear from the above that one product of the sustained attention to cognitive factors in psychopathology and psychotherapy has been the differentiation, both subtle and obvious, between various forms of cognitive therapy. Mahoney (1988) has recently enumerated 17 subtypes of cognitive therapy, ranging from early formulations such as personal construct therapy, logotherapy, and rational-emotive therapy, through intermediate formulations such as Lazarus's multimodal therapy and the problem-solving therapies, to the recent constructivist cognitive therapy and cognitive-developmental therapy. Safran's cognitive-interpersonal approach (Safran & Segal, 1990) should also be added to this list as a recent development in cognitive therapy. Dobson (1988) has categorized the various forms of cognitive therapy as involving covert conditioning models, information-processing models, cognitive learning models, and structural models. The more recent theoretical developments that guide cognitive interventions are of particular interest because they provide explicit models for maintaining flexibility, addressing interpersonal issues, and targeting structural change. For these reasons particular attention will be given to these recent models in this chapter.

A historical context is helpful in gaining an appreciation of the similarities and differences between the various forms of cognitive therapy that are currently practiced. The development of cognitive therapies follows an "evolutionary" path that fits nicely with Kuhn's notions of scientific revolutions and paradigm shifts (Kuhn, 1962). Several important historical developments are noteworthy. These developments were temporally sequenced in such a way as to account for the recent distinction between what are called rationalist-based and constructivist-based perspectives on cognitive therapy (Guidano & Liotti, 1983; Mahoney, 1985). In contrasting rationalist and constructivist perspectives it is important not to view them as mutually exclusive. The value in drawing a distinction between them is that the therapeutic interventions that derive from each perspective can be explicated. Researchers and therapists can then evaluate the conditions under which adopting each conceptual perspective (and therefore the types of interventions that follow) is most appropriate at a given time for a given therapeutic target. Prior to discussing these perspectives, however, several important developmental milestones in the growth of cognitive therapy will be noted.

## Behavior Analysis and Therapy

Much of current cognitive therapy practice has its base in behavior analysis and therapy. These, for the main part, are Dobson's (1988) covert conditioning models, which became popular in the late 1960s and early 1970s. Two events are important here. First, operant conditioning techniques were applied to covert events directly (see Mahoney, 1974). Techniques such as covert conditioning (Cautela, 1966) and thought stopping (Wolpe, 1969) illustrate this stage of development. Second,  Bandura's social learning theory (Bandura, 1976) legitimized phenomena such as observational learning and other nonbehavioral mechanisms (e.g., self-efficacy; Bandura, 1977). Essential contributions by Meichenbaum in developing self-instructional training (Meichenbaum, 1977), D'Zurilla and Goldfried in their work on problem-solving therapy and cognitive restructuring (D'Zurilla & Goldfried, 1971) and Rehm in developing self-control therapy (Rehm, 1981) are also important to note.

These forms of cognitive therapy, which developed from behavioral models, are characterized by being highly structured, didactic, and educational in nature. Relatively little attention is given to the therapeutic relationship or to the therapeutic process. For instance, Rehm's self-control therapy focuses on three cognitive processes: self-monitoring, self-evaluation, and self-reinforcement (Rehm, 1981). Treatment is directed specifically to these processes. For self-monitoring, Rehm proposes that depressives attend to negative relative to positive information, and that they attend more to short- than to long-term consequences. Patients are instructed about these processes, and strategies for altering them are taught and practiced. Similarly, problems in self-evaluation are thought to reflect overly stringent standards for evaluation and negative self-attribution, and patients learn specific strategies for correcting these problems. Finally, patients are taught self-reinforcement strategies, since lack of self-reinforcement is considered a component of the depressive reaction. The educational focus reflected in self-control therapy is characteristic also of Meichenbaum's stress-inoculation training (Meichenbaum, 1977). Meichenbaum's protocol is highly structured and involves distinct education, skills acquisition (relaxation, attention diversion, and self-instructional training), and application (exposure) phases.

While there are data that clearly document the efficacy of these therapy protocols (see Meichenbaum, 1977; Rehm, 1981), they have not received widespread clinical application. This may in part relate to the fact that such treatments were not developed in the context of a clinical practice and tended to be theoretically pure. Much of the validation work was conducted on nonclinical or subclinical populations, which limits ecological validity and generalizability.

## *Rational-Emotive Therapy and Beck's Cognitive Therapy*

Another important developmental milestone in cognitive therapy is represented by the work of Albert Ellis and Aaron Beck. Their models of cognitive therapy (rational-emotive therapy and cognitive therapy, respectively) were developed separately from the behavioral approaches, and in Ellis's case predated them. It is noteworthy that Ellis and Beck developed their models in the context of clinical practice. As a result, their therapies can be seen as forms of psychotherapy, as opposed to the more theoretical cognitive-behavioral modification programs.

While Ellis's rational-emotive therapy (RET) and Beck's cognitive therapy are based on shared theoretical notions, there are procedural differences between the two that are important to note. Rational-emotive therapy tends to be more didactic than Socratic. Patients are encouraged to adopt the A-B-C model of distress (activating event-belief-consequences) in which belief is primary. Therapist interventions focus on directing patients to attend to their "irrational beliefs," to recognize them as irrational, and to give them up by debating, discriminating (wants from needs, desires from demands), and disputing (see Ellis & Greiger, 1977, for more details). Beck's cognitive therapy (Beck, 1976), on the other hand, tends to be more Socratic than didactic, and therapists' interventions are generally less forceful. Greater attention is placed on experiential learning. In Beck's approach, therapists encourage patients to monitor their own experience, identify dysfunctional cognitions (*automatic thoughts* is the buzzword in cognitive therapy), test them out, and draw their own conclusions, rather than point out irrational beliefs and actively (sometimes vehemently) dispute them with the patient, as in RET.

The publication of the text *Cognitive Therapy of Depression* by Beck and his colleagues (Beck, Rush, Shaw, & Emery, 1979) proved to be a seminal contribution to the field, in part because it was written as a therapy manual. By integrating theoretical notions (e.g., negative cognitive triad, distorted perceptual processes, dsyfunctional assumptions) and intervention techniques (e.g., mastery-pleasure exercises, evidence gathering, cognitive restructuring), Beck *et al.* (1979) provided a structure for therapy that facilitated clinically based evaluation. This has done much to advance the recent trend within psychotherapy research toward clearer specification of treatment variables and evaluation of therapists' actual in-session behavior (Williams & Spitzer, 1984).

Beck's cognitive therapy is specific enough to allow therapy to be operationalized and evaluated (e.g., sessions are structured by agenda setting, problem exploration and intervention, summary, and homework assignment) and flexible enough to accommodate patients' current needs. The value of this particular model of cognitive therapy is illustrated in the recent National Institute of Mental Health's (NIMH) Treatment of Depression Collaborative Research Progam (TDCRP; Elkin *et al.*, 1985). In this study, considerable effort was devoted to developing clear standards and evaluation criteria for the training and monitoring of therapists' actual behavior within psychotherapy (cognitive and interpersonal therapies) sessions (Rounsaville, Chevron, & Weissmann, 1984; Shaw, 1984).

## The Integrationist Movement

A relatively recent development that has had significant influence on the practice of cognitive therapy is the integration of noncognitive theoretical models with cognitive models. This represents another developmental milestone for cognitive therapy and reflects the general trend toward theoretical integration in psychotherapy (e.g., Goldfried, 1982; note also the recent development of the Society for the Exploration of Psychotherapy Integration).

Several cognitive theorists have integrated the cognitive model with Kelly's personal construct theory (Neimeyer *et al.*, 1985), Bowlby's attachment theory (Bolwby, 1985), Sullivan's interpersonal theory (Crowley, 1985; Safran & Segal, 1990), and even (although not given great attention) Adlerian psychotherapy (Shulman, 1985). Accompanying this trend has been the integration of cognitive psychology into the mainstream of cognitive therapy. This is illustrated best by the growing body of research on the role of schemata in cognition and in psychopathology (see Hollon & Kriss, 1984; Kuiper & Olinger, 1986; Turk & Salovey, 1985a, 1985b).

Integrating noncognitive with cognitive models has led to shifts in the therapeutic targets as well as the therapeutic process of cognitive therapy. The most well-articulated shifts are illustrated by the work of Guidano and Liotti (1983) and Mahoney (1988) on the constructivist-developmental approach to cognitive therapy and by Safran's (Safran & Segal, 1990) work on the cognitive-interpersonal approach to cognitive therapy. Each of these models will now be addressed.

*The Constructivist-Developmental Approach to Cognitive Therapy*

Guidano and Liotti (1983) provide an excellent model of a constructivist-developmental approach to cognitive therapy. Their approach relies heavily on developmental theory and structural models of knowledge. They differentiate tacit from explicit knowing and highlight the central role of self-knowledge in emotional dysfunction and well-being. Attachment is seen as playing a major role in the development of self-knowledge. Guidano and Liotti (among others, such as Safran, Vallis, Segal, and Shaw, 1986, and Meichenbaum and Gilmore, 1984) differentiate core from peripheral cognitive events. Core cognitive events are defined as being central to the experience of the self, whereas peripheral cognitive events are noncentral (see Safran *et al.*, 1986). As such, changes in core cognitive processes are thought to lead to greater and more lasting clinical change.

Guidano and Liotti (1983) highlight therapeutic interventions designed to alter deep, core structure (which they refer to as the metaphysical hard core). Techniques such as cognitive restructuring or gathering evidence are seen as affecting peripheral, but not necessarily deep, cognitive structures. Change in deep structure requires an in-depth examination of the developmental stages leading to the formation of deep structure self-knowledge. Thus, the therapists influenced by these notions spend extensive amounts of time on historical and process-focused issues, relative to therapists focused on problem solving and symptom resolution.

Mahoney (1988), who also supports a constructivist-developmental model of cognitive therapy, draws a distinction between what he terms rationalist approaches to cognitive therapy and developmental-constructivist approaches. In distinguishing these approaches he highlights differences in the conceptualization of the nature of reality (ontology) as well as assumptions regarding the nature of knowledge and the process of change (epistemology).

According to Mahoney (1988), the rationalist view is that reality is external and stable, something that can be confirmed and validated. In contrast, within the constructivist view, reality is subjective and idiosyncratic. Although this distinction appears clear from a philosophical perspective, it is less clear whether it distinguishes among different forms of cognitive therapy (e.g., Meichenbaum's self-instructional training and Beck's cognitive therapy from Guidano and Liotti's constructivist cognitive therapy). Mahoney asserts that Beck's and Ellis's models are influenced primarily by the rationalist perspective. However, Beck has clearly maintained that reality is a subjective experience, dependent on the appraisal of the individual. Similarly, inherent in Ellis's A-B-C model is the role of subjective beliefs. It is the case, however, that the models of Beck and Ellis emphasize that there is a reality of sorts, one that serves as an objective standard which, when appealed to, can alter dysfunctional appraisal processes. The notions of collecting *data* and appealing to the *evidence* to correct cognitive *distortions* follow from this view of reality as a validating referent. In contrast, Guidano and Liotti's and Mahoney's models place more emphasis on the active creation of reality in a feed-forward fashion (see Mahoney's discussion of sensory metatheories versus motor metatheories of the mind). Thus, relative differences in the view of reality can be found between therapy models influenced by rationalist perspectives (Beck's and Ellis's models) and those influenced by constructivist perspectives (Guidano and Liotti's and Mahoney's models).

Mahoney also makes important distinctions between rationalist and constructivist perspectives with respect to the nature of knowledge and the process of change. According to a rationalist perspective, knowledge is validated by logic and reason, with priority given to thought over emotion. The notion of controlling emotions by controlling thoughts follows from this. In contrast, constructivism maintains that knowledge is an integrated cognitive-behavioral-affective experience. Rationalist and constructivist perspectives also differ in their notions of human change. From a rationalist perspective, change proceeds according to cause-and-effect relationships, characterized by associationism. From a constructivist perspective, however, change involves structural differentiation, where mental representations are transformed and refined in an evolutionary fashion (Mahoney, 1988).

## The Cognitive-Interpersonal Approach to Cognitive Therapy

Another recent theoretical development that has stimulated adaptation in cognitive therapy is illustrated by Safran's work on cognitive-interpersonal approaches (Safran 1984a, 1984b, 1988; Safran & Segal, 1990). Safran emphasizes the interpersonal nature of an individual's functioning and distress and has developed therapeutic interventions directed toward facilitating change, at a core level, in interpersonal schemata. An interpersonal schema is "a generic cognitive representation of interpersonal events" (p. 5) that is "abstracted on the basis of interactions with attachment figures and . . . permits the individual to predict interactions in a way that increases the probability of maintaining relatedness with these figures . . . " (p. 13, Safran, 1988). Safran is clearly introducing a new and integrative notion here, and much of his recent work has been in the development of cognitive-interpersonal interventions (see Safran & Segal, 1990).

An important aspect of Safran's work is his distinction between the information-processing model and the ecological model of cognitive functioning. Well known to cognitive theorists and therapists, the information-processing model posits that individuals receive and transform information in a somewhat isolated and relatively passive manner (the computer analogy). The emphasis in the information-processing model is on the processing of incoming information, not on the individual's role in acting on the environment. The ecological model, on the other hand, advocates that individuals need to be studied in the context of their real-world environment, which is by and large interpersonal. Further, according to the ecological model, knowing and acting are intrinsically connected (thereby rendering irrelevant the cognition-affect primacy debate; Lazarus, 1984; Zajonc, 1984), and psychological processes need to be seen from a functional perspective (see Safran & Segal, 1990). As expected, these theoretical principles influence the therapist's approach. For example, considerable therapeutic value, both in terms of understanding the patient and intervening on dysfunctional interpersonal processes, can be gained by focused attention on the patient-therapist interaction and its relationship to the patient's distress and self-schemata.

In summary, current cognitive therapy has been marked by a series of developmental stages. Historically, behavioral analysis and therapy was applied to covert events. Beck then integrated many of these behavioral and cognitive-behavioral developments into his model of cognitive therapy, which is perhaps the most widely accepted approach to cognitive therapy (although some might argue that this distinction belongs to Ellis). Currently, Beck's model is being intergrated with other theoretical ideas, most notably constructivist-developmental and cognitive-interpersonal principles. This is leading to a departure in how cognitive therapy is being implemented clinically. This is not to imply that the cognitive therapies influenced by the rationalist perspective are less appropriate than they once were. Recent theoretical developments should be considered evolutionary, not revolutionary. What is needed is a way of evaluating the conditions under which the different conceptual perspectives of cognitive therapy (and the interventions that follow from these conceptualizations) are more or less appropriate to given populations and/or cases. In an attempt to facilitate this, the remainder of this chapter is devoted to elaborating on the practical implications of distinguishing cognitive therapy guided by the rationalist perspective from cognitive therapy guided by the constructivist-developmental-interpersonal (constructivist, for short) perspective. In doing so, I am not advocating that the two perspectives are mutually exclusive. It is the integration of the two perspectives that is likely to lead to the most flexible and effective form of cognitive therapy. However, the clear specification of these differences is required in order to guide the research and clinical exposure necessary to evaluate the incremental validity of the recent theoretical developments.

## Practical Consequences of the Rationalist-Constructivist Dichotomy

The theoretical model or conceptual framework explicitly or implicitly endorsed by the therapist will necessarily guide the choice of interventions and clinical phenomena that are addressed in therapy (see Shaw, 1984; Chapter 2, this volume). Given the distinction between the rationalist and constructivist perspectives, therefore, one can contrast the nature of the cognitive therapy that would be conducted by following each of these theoretical approaches.

To understand the extent of these differences it is helpful to draw the distinction between cognitive content, cognitive process, and cognitive structure (Hollon & Kriss, 1984; Segal, 1990; Turk & Salovey, 1985a, 1985b). *Cognitive content* refers to the accessible thoughts and images experienced by an individual. This material can be accessed by direct inquiry (e.g., "What was going through your mind when you felt your mood drop suddenly?"), assuming that patients report their cognitions candidly. *Cognitive process* refers to the ways in which information is acted upon during construal. It is here where the notion of cognitive distortions arises (Beck *et al.*, 1979). Beck has enumerated a variety of distorting processes relevant to emotional distress, including selective abstraction (where only part of available information is attended to), arbitrary inference (jumping to conclusions), and all-or-nothing thinking (the tendency to draw extreme conclusions and ignore ambiguity). Finally, *cognitive structure* refers to nonconscious schemata, which are affectively charged meaning structures that are hierarchically organized (see Safran *et al.*, 1986). These structures guide the overall processing of information (i.e., cognitive processes and cognitive content). It has generally been accepted that not all cognitions (automatic thoughts or dysfunctional schemata) are equally important. Some processes are regarded as more important (central or core) and others less important (peripheral) (Arnkoff, 1980; Guidano & Liotti, 1983; Safran *et al.*, 1986).

With these distinctions in mind, therapists would be expected to focus more on cognitive content and process than cognitive structure when following a rationalist-based perspective. This would follow from a view of knowledge as being validated by logic and reason, with priority given to thought over emotion (change the way you think and this will change the way you feel). In contrast, therapists who adopt a constructivist-based perspective would be expected to focus more on cognitive structure than cognitive content or process. Thus, cognitive therapy applied according to a rationalist perspective tends to be content focused, structured, and oriented toward education and skills acquisition. It is instructive to examine the cognitive therapy of depression of Beck *et al.* (1979) in light of the rationalist-constructivist distinction. Beck's model is a useful protocol to examine because of its popularity, demonstrated efficacy, and flexibility. Further, although Beck *et al.* (1979) tend to be content focused, they clearly stress the importance of the therapeutic relationship and nonspecific factors (see Vallis *et al.*, 1988) in therapy.

Beck's cognitive model of depression is built around the negative cognitive triad, faulty information-processing styles, and dysfunctional self-referent assumptions. Therapy is highly structured, and much of the therapist's behavior involves educating patients as to the role of cognitions in distress and in recognizing and connecting the kinds of thinking errors characteristic of their disorder. Treatment is focused around patients' acquisition of relevant behavioral skills (mastery and pleasure exercises, graded task performance, role playing and rehearsal) and cognitive skills (examining available evidence, reattribution, generating alternatives, recording and reappraising negative cognitions) to overcome their cognitive distortions. The patient and therapist keep detailed notes, negotiate a structured agenda, routinely evaluate homework, and spend time rating the patient's degree of belief in negative cognitions and current affect (such ratings form the basis of evaluations of cognitive therapy; see Persons & Burns, 1985). The initial phase of therapy focuses on symptom reduction through exploration of cognitive content and education. Later, the therapist focuses on dysfunctional beliefs, which relate conceptually to structural schemata. Schemata-based interventions include examining the advantages and disadvantages of dysfunctional beliefs and practicing behaviors inconsistent with the dysfunctional belief. Burns's (1980) self-help manual entitled *Feeling Good: The New Mood Therapy* is an excellent illustration of the technical focus of cognitive therapy. Thus, while not exclusively so, Beck's protocol-based approach to cognitive therapy can be seen to be guided heavily by the rationalist-based perspective of cognition and therapeutic change.

In contrast to therapy based on the rationalist perspective, therapy based on the constructivist model is more focused on cognitive structure and its development, within the context of the therapeutic relationship. As noted earlier, Guidano and Liotti (1983) illustrate this approach clearly. Their approach is less didactic, structured, and educational than that of Beck *et al.* (1979), Meichenbaum (1977), or Rehm (1981). While symptom relief is sought, it is not, initially at least, the primary focus. Instead, therapy is oriented toward the identification of core organizing schemata. Therapists spend a great deal of their time trying to understand the patients phenomenology vis-à-vis these core schemata (deep structure versus surface structure; Arnkoff, 1980). Therapists' interventions are likely to be less distinctive than those deriving from a rationalist perspective. Therapists work to help patients come to appreciate (not learn) how they see themselves and how this view influences their distress. This is done in an experiential fashion (see Guidano & Liotti, 1983; Mahoney, 1988; Safran & Segal, 1990). Considerable emphasis is placed on decentering (being able to observe one's own thought processes and appreciate their impact), as opposed to development of specific coping strategies (e.g., record keeping, disputing negative automatic thoughts, using "flash cards"; see Young & Beck, 1982). Further, in following a constructivist perspective, cognitive therapists would explore the patient's developmental context in greater detail. Such a focus is designed to aid in identifying core dysfunctional beliefs and the decentering process. Thus, more weight is given to the process of therapy than to intervention techniques.

Therapists guided by constructivist notions often use their own relationship with the patient in therapy to a greater extent than therapists guided by rationalist notions (Jacobson, 1989; Safran & Segal, 1990). As a consequence of the therapist's conceptualization, constructivist-based cognitive therapy tends to be more flexible and more integrated with noncognitive therapies than rationalist-based cognitive therapy. However, it runs the risk of being a less distinctive form of therapy.

A brief case example may be useful to further illustrate how the rationalist and constructivist conceptualizations differentially influence treatment. A married, 49-year-old female lawyer (D.A.) was referred to the author for treatment of anxiety. D.A. had a 20-year history of agoraphobic fears and was housebound at one point. However, at the time of referral she was functioning quite well. She experienced relatively few panic attacks and was able to maintain her job and household responsibilities with relative ease. She was seeking help in order to eliminate the remaining anxiety associated with extended travel (e.g., greater than 20 miles from her home).

Adopting a rationalist conceptualization, the therapist may have encouraged D.A. to expose herself, in a graded fashion, to anxiety-precipitating events, such as extended travel, and to record her automatic thoughts and behavioral avoidance tendencies. Cognitive (rational reappraisal, self-instructions) and behavioral (exposure to facilitate habituation, relaxation) interventions could be implemented to reduce avoidance and physiological reactivity and to increase self-efficacy.

Adopting a constructivist conceptualization, which the therapist did in this case, led to a different treatment approach. Rather than help D.A. develop greater control over her anxiety, the therapist observed that the patient was functioning well and was repeatedly able to cope with anxious situations without avoidance and hypothesized that further increasing her self-control might leave her vulnerable to future anxiety. Any prospect of being out of control elicited thoughts of weakness, inferiority, and anticipated rejection. Further, the experience of physiological arousal was interpreted as loss of control. To increase D.A.'s ability to control might be calming (peripheral change), but it would leave her vulnerable to situations involving normal anxiety, such as distress associated with an ill relative or witnessing a traffic accident (stressful events which had recently occurred in her life). Such uncontrollable situations were associated with increased symptomatology. It is also interesting to note that repeated attempts at relaxation training consistently elicited panic attacks. She viewed relaxing as giving up control.

Rather than adopting a problem-solving approach, the therapist explored the issue of control and targeted the patient's beliefs that she must be in control at all times and that physiological arousal was a sign of loss of control. The meaning of loss of control was explored in light of her developmental background (she was placed in a foster home at age 10 due to mother's emotional problems) and current life circumstances (her husband had had a recent heart attack, and she was the primary breadwinner). Using this approach, D.A. was able to see how seeking excessive control was dysfunctional (i.e., decentering and reappraisal followed experiential exploration of her cognitive style). Her distress greatly decreased once she allowed herself to be more spontaneous in her emotional experience and expression.

Clearly, cognitive therapists currently face a number of choices concerning conceptual models and intervention strategies. What is needed is a mechanism by which therapists can make informed judgments concerning the circumstances in which one approach is more appropriate than another (see Chapter 2, this volume). If D.A. had presented with frequent panic attacks, poor self-efficacy, and extensive avoidance, following a more rationalist-based perspective may have been more desirable. Ideally, one could envision a decision-tree in which certain patient characteristics or processes rule in or rule out particular conceptual and technical approaches. Unfortunately, we have not yet reached this stage. Currently, it is most important to clearly differentiate the existing cognitive perspectives so that the appropiate research can follow.

## Implications of Rationalist and Constructivist Perspectives on Cognitive Therapy

Rationalist-based and constructivist-based perspectives have implications for the future practice of cognitive therapy. The main areas that warrant consideration in this regard are research, training, and therapy integration.

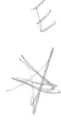

With respect to *research*, the cognitive therapies influenced by the rationalist perspective would be expected to lend themselves more easily to testability. Again, Beck's cognitive therapy is most illustrative of this. There is a clear treatment manual that provides a session-by-session outline of the course of cognitive therapy, as well as a compendium of cognitive therapy interventions. This has led to the development of rating scales to evaluate therapist adherence to the protocol and competence in implementing cognitive therapy. Hollon and his colleagues, as part of the NIMH Treatment of Depression Collaborative

Research Program, developed the Collaborative Study Psychotherapy Rating Scale to assess therapist behavior (see DeRubeis, Hollon, Evans, & Bemis, 1982). This group has been able to use the scale to clearly differentiate between therapists performing Beck *et al.*'s (1979) cognitive therapy, interpersonal therapy (IPT; Klerman, Weissman, Rounsaville, & Chevron, 1984), and pharmacotherapy plus clinical management. Similarly, within the same Treatment of Depression Collaborative Research Program, Shaw and his colleagues (Dobson, Shaw, & Vallis, 1985; Vallis, Shaw, & Dobson, 1986) have used Young and Beck's (1980) Cognitive Therapy Scale to evaluate therapist competency. The CTS items rely heavily on evaluating the technical aspects of cognitive therapy, and the ratings were used in the training of the NIMH therapists. Meichenbaum's stress inoculation training and Rehm's (1981) self-control therapy, also heavily influenced by a rationalist perspective, are further examples of forms of cognitive therapy well suited to research methodologies emphasizing operationalization and standardization.

In contrast, cognitive therapy guided by the constructivist perspective appears to be more difficult to evaluate, particularly within a comparative or outcome-oriented paradigm. Specifically, technique becomes more difficult to identify and evaluate in constructivist applications of cognitive therapy. One could predict that constructivist-based cognitive therapy would be less distinct from noncognitive therapy than rationalist-based cognitive therapy. This could be evaluated by comparing rationalist-based and constructivist-based cognitive therapy to noncognitive therapy, using scales such as the Collaborative Study Psychotherapy Rating Scale or the Cognitive Therapy Scale. Regardless of the outcome of such comparisons, whether less distinctiveness is advantageous (in that constructivist-based cognitive therapy may be closer to a wholistic approach), disadvantageous (in that essential techniques are watered down; see Goldfied, 1988; Shaw, 1988; Shulman, 1988; Strupp, 1988), or simply more complex (in that technique becomes more difficult to assess) remains to be seen.

It should be noted that while cognitive therapy guided by a constructivist perspective may be more difficult to evaluate with a research design focused on operationalizing interventions, standardizing treatment, and comparing treatments based on unique features, it may be well suited for the research paradigm proposed by Rice and Greenberg (1984). In this paradigm, psychotherapy change process is evaluated in a microscopic fashion (i.e., using in-session critical incidents as the units of analysis).

Another area in which the rationalist-constructivist distinction may influence the practice of cognitive therapy is in the area of *training*.

Rationalist-based cognitive therapy lends itself to training in a highly behavioral and programmatic manner. The relevant technical interventions can be dismantled from the overall treatment, modeled, and rehearsed. Further, the theoretical constructs necessary to understand and implement rationalist-based cognitive therapy can be clearly and easily identified and articulated. Constructivist-based cognitive therapy lends itself less well to this form of training. It may be that rationalist-based cognitive therapy is more suited to graduate-level training, where therapists are struggling for a clear model of what to do, when, and why. Constructivist-based cognitive therapy, on the other hand, may be better suited to more experienced therapists, comfortable with flexibility and well informed about systems of therapy and models of psychotherapy change.

Finally, rationalist-based and constructivist-based perspectives on cognitive therapy lend themselves differently to *integration* with other forms of psychotherapy. Constructivist-based perspectives are more easily integrated with noncognitive therapies, both conceptually and technically. Conceptually, within constructivist perspectives cognition is explicitly integrated with affective and developmental processes. Technically, constructivist-oriented therapists are explicitly encouraged to combine cognitive with noncognitive techniques such as the Gestalt two-chair technique or the psychodynamic focus on the "transference." Rationalist-based perspectives on cognitive therapy, on the other hand, emphasize cognitive therapy's distinctiveness from, rather than its similarities to, noncognitive therapies.

## SUMMARY

I have attempted in this chapter to trace the development of cognitive therapy and to emphasize the current diversity in approaches. It is important to reiterate the value, both demonstrated and potential, of both the rationalist-based and constructivist-based perspectives in providing conceptual guidelines for implementing cognitive therapy. Rationalist and constructivist perspectives are complementary and afford maximum flexibility. It is truly an exciting time for cognitive therapy and cognitive therapists. Cognitive therapists are now in a position to deal with issues that once posed difficulty. For instance, early formulations of cognitive therapy implicitly endorsed a unidimensional view of emotion. Emotions were the products of cognition and were to be controlled. Greenberg and Safran (1987) have challenged this view by making a tripartite distinction between primary emotions, secondary emotions, and instrumental emotions. Incorporating such a distinction into the practice of cognitive therapy allows for a more flexible and, it is hoped, effective approach (e.g., it provides a rationale by which some emotions [secondary emotions] are important to control, whereas others [primary emotions] are important not to control). As well, by integrating rationalist and constructivist perspectives, cognitive therapy should become more adaptable to populations other than those with unipolar depressive disorders and anxiety disorders. The purpose of this text is to outline how cognitive therapy can be applied to nontraditional populations, such as personality-disordered patients, medical patients, or those suffering from posttraumatic stress disorder.

# REFERENCES

Arnkoff, D. (1980). Psychotherapy from the perspective of cognitive theory. In M. Mahoney (Ed.), *Psychotherapy process* (pp. 339-361). New York: Plenum.

Bandura, A. (1976). *Social learning theory.* Englewood Cliffs, NJ: Prentice Hall.

Bandura, A. (1977). Self-efficacy: Toward a unifying theory of behavioral change. *Psychological Review, 84,* 191-215.

Beck, A. T. (1976). *Cognitive therapy and the emotional disorders.* New York: International Universities Press.

Beck, A. T. (1983). Cognitive therapy of depression: New perspectives. In P. Clayton & J. Barrett, *New approaches* (pp. 265-290). New York: Rowan Press.

Beck, A. T. (1985). Cognitive therapy, behavior therapy, psychoanalysis, and pharmacotherapy: A cognitive continuum. In M. Mahoney & A. Freeman (Eds.), *Cognition and psychotherapy* (pp. 325-347). New York: Plenum.

Beck, A. T., Rush, A. J., Shaw, B., & Emery, G. (1979). *Cognitive therapy of depression.* New York: Guilford.

Bowlby, J. (1985). The role of childhood experience in cognitive disturbance. In M. Mahoney & A. Freeman (Eds.), *Cognition and psychotherapy* (pp. 181-200). New York: Plenum.

Burns, D. (1980). *Feeling good: The new mood therapy.* New York: William Morrow.

Cautela, J. (1966). Treatment of compulsive behavior by covert sensitization. *Psychological Record, 16,* 33-41.

Coyne, J., & Gotlib, I. (1983). The role of cognitions in depression. A critical appraisal. *Psychological Bulletin, 94,* 472-505.

Crowley, R. (1985). Cognition in interpersonal theory and practice. In M. Mahoney & A. Freeman (Eds.), *Cognition and psychotherapy* (pp. 291-312). New York: Plenum.

DeRubeis, R., Hollon, S., Evans, M., & Bemis, K. (1982). Can psychotherapies for depression be discriminated? A systematic investigation of cognitive therapy and interpersonal therapy. *Journal of Consulting and Clinical Psychology, 50,* 744-756.

Dobson, K. (1988). *Handbook of cognitive-behavioral therapies.* New York: Guilford.

Dobson, K., Shaw, B., & Vallis, T. M. (1985). The reliability of competency ratings on cognitive-behavior therapists. *British Journal of Clinical Psychology, 24,* 295-300.

D'Zurilla, T., & Goldfried, M. (1971). Problem-solving and behavior modification. *Journal of Abnormal Psychology, 78,* 107-126.

Elkin, I., Parloff, M., Hadley, S., & Autry, J. (1985). NIMH treatment of depression collaborative research program: Background and research plan. *Archives of General Psychiatry, 42,* 305-316.

Ellis, A. (1977). The basic clinical theory of rational-emotive therapy. In A. Ellis & R. Grieger (Eds.), *Handbook of rational-emotive therapy* (pp. 3-34). New York: Springer.

Ellis, A., & Grieger, R. (1977). *Handbook of rational-emotive therapy.* New York: Springer.

Frank, J. D. (1985). Therapeutic components shared by all psychotherapies. In M. J. Mahoney & A. Freeman (Eds.), *Cognition and psychotherapy* (pp. 49-80). New York: Plenum.

Goldfried, M. (1982). *Converging themes in psychotherapy: Trends in psychodynamic, humanistic and behavioral practise* New York: Springer.

Goldfried, M. (1988). A comment on therapeutic change: A response. *Journal of Cognitive Psychotherapy: An International Quarterly, 2,* 9-93.

Greenberg, L., & Safran, J. (1987). *Emotions in psychotherapy.* New York: Guilford.

Guidano, V., & Liotti, G. (1983). *Cognitive processes and emotional disorders: A structural approach to psychotherapy.* New York: Guilford.

Hollon, S., & Kriss, M. (1984). Cognitive factors in clinical research and practice. *Clinical Psychology Review 4,* 35-76.

Jacobson, N. S. (1989). The therapist-client relationship in cognitive behavior therapy: Implications for treating depression. *Journal of Cognitive Psychotherapy: An International Quarterly, 3,* 85-96.

Klerman, G., Weissman, M., Rounsaville, B., & Chevron, E. (1984). *Interpersonal psychotherapy of depression.* New York: Basic Books.

Kovacs, M., & Beck, A. T. (1978). Maladaptive cognitive structures in depression. *American Journal of Psychiatry, 135,* 525-533.

Kuhn, T. (1962). *The structure of scientific revolution.* Chicago: University of Chicago Press.

Kuiper, N., & Olinger, J. (1986). Dysfunctional attitudes and a self-worth contingency model of depression. In P. Kendall (Ed.), *Advances in cognitive-behavioral research and therapy* (Vol. 5). New York: Academic Press.

Lazarus, R. (1984). On the primacy of cognition. *American Psychologist, 39,* 124-129.

Mahoney, M. (1974). *Cognition and behavior modification.* New York: Ballinger.

Mahoney, M. (1985). Psychotherapy and human change processes. In M. Mahoney & A. Freeman (Eds.), *Cognition and psychotherapy* (pp. 3-48). New York: Plenum.

Mahoney, M. (1988). The cognitive sciences and psychotherapy: Patterns in a developing relationship. In K. Dobson (Ed.), *Handbook of cognitive-behavior therapies* (pp. 357-386). New York: Guilford.

Mahoney, M., & Freeman, A. (1985). *Cognition and psychotherapy.* New York: Plenum.

Matarazzo, R., Philips, J., Weins, A., & Saslow, G. (1965). Learning the art of interviewing: A study of what beginning students do and their pattern of change. *Psychotherapy: Theory, Research and Practice, 2,* 49-60.

Meichenbaum, D. (1977). *Cognitive-behavior modification.* New York: Plenum.

Meichenbaum, D., & Gilmore, B. (1984). The nature of unconscious processes: A cognitive-behavioral perspective. In K. S. Bowers & D. Meichenbaum (Eds.), *The unconscious reconsidered.* New York: Wiley.

Neimeyer, R., Twentyman, C., & Prezant, D. (1985). Cognitive and interpersonal group therapies for depression: A progress report. *The Cognitive Behaviorist, 7*(1), 21-22.

Persons, J., & Burns, D. (1985). Mechanisms of action of cognitive therapy. The relative contribution of technical and interpersonal interventions. *Cognitive Therapy and Research, 9,* 539-552.

Persons, J., & Burns, D., & Perloff, J. M. (1988). Predictors of dropout and outcome in cognitive therapy for depression in a private practice setting. *Cognitive Therapy and Research, 12,* 557-576.

Primakoff, L., Epstein, N., & Covi, L. (1989). Homework compliance: An uncontrolled variable in cognitive therapy outcome research. In W. Dryden & P. Trower (Eds.), *Cognitive psychotherapy: Stasis and change* (pp. 175-189). New York: Springer.

Rehm, L. (1981). A self-control therapy program for treatment of depression. In T. Clarkin & H. Glazer (Eds.), *Depression: Behavioral and directive intervention strategies* (pp. 68-110). New York: Garland.

Rice, L., & Greenberg, L. (1984). *Patterns of change.* New York: Guilford.

Riskind, J., & Steer, R. (1984). Do maladaptive attitudes cause depression: Misconceptions of cognitive theory. *Archives of General Psychiatry, 41,* 1111.

Rounsaville, B., Chevron, E., & Weissman, M. (1984). Specification of techniques in interpersonal psychotherapy. In T. Williams and R. Spitzer (Eds.), *Psychotherapy research: Where are we and where should we go?* New York: Guilford.

Rush, A. J., & Giles, D. (1982). Cognitive therapy: Theory and research. In A. J. Rush (Ed.), *Short-term psychotherapies for depression* (pp. 143-181). New York: Guilford.

Safran, J. D. (1984a). Assessing the cognitive-interpersonal cycle. *Cognitive Therapy and Research, 8,* 333-348.

Safran, J. D. (1984b). Some implications of Sullivan's interpersonal theory for cognitive therapy. In M. Reda & M. Mahoney (Eds.), *Cognitive psychotherapies: Recent developments in theory, research and practice.* Cambridge, MA: Ballinger.

Safran, J. D. (1988). *A refinement of cognitive behavioural theory and practise in light of interpersonal theory.* Clarke Institute of Psychiatry, Toronto.

Safran, J. D., & Segal, Z. V. (1990). *Cognitive therapy: An interpersonal process perspective.* New York: Basic Books.

Safran, J. D., Vallis, T. M., Segal, Z. V., & Shaw, B. F. (1986). Assessment of core cognitive processes in cognitive therapy. *Cognitive Therapy and Research, 10,* 509-526.

Segal, Z. V. (1990). Appraisal of the self-schema construct in cognitive models of depression. *Psychological Bulletin, 103,* 147-162.

Shaw, B. F. (1984). Specification of the training and evaluation of cognitive therapists for outcome studies. In J. Williams & R. Spitzer (Eds.), *Psychotherapy research: Where are we and where should we go?* New York: Guilford.

Shaw, B. F. (1988). The value of researching psychotherapy techniques: A response. *Journal of Cognitive Psychotherapy: An International Quarterly, 2,* 83-87.

Shaw, B. F., & Segal, Z. V. (1989). Introduction to cognitive theory and therapy. In A. Frances & R. Holes (Eds.), *Review of psychiatry, Volume 7* (pp. 538-553). New York: American Psychiatric Press.

Shulman, B. (1985). Cognitive therapy and the individual psychology of Alfred Adler. In M. Mahoney & A. Freeman (Eds.), *Cognition and psychotherapy* (pp. 243-258). New York: Plenum.

Shulman, B. (1988). Dissecting the elements of therapeutic change: A response. *Journal of Cognitive Psychotherapy: An International Quarterly, 2,* 95-103.

Silverman, J., Silverman, J., & Eardley, D. (1984). Do maladaptive attitudes cause depression? *Archives of General Psychiatry, 41,* 28-30.

Simons, A., Garfield, S., & Murphy, G. (1984). The process of change in cognitive therapy and pharmacotherapy for depression: Changes in mood and cognition. *Archives of General Psychiatry, 41,* 45-51.

Strupp, H. (1988). What is therapeutic change? *Journal of Cognitive Psychotherapy: An International Quarterly, 2,* 75-82.

Turk, D., & Salovey, P. (1985a). Cognitive structures, cognitive processes, and cognitive-behavior modification: I. Client issues. *Cognitive Therapy and Research, 9,* 1-18.

Turk, D., & Salovey, P. (1985b). Cognitive structures, cognitive processes, and cognitive-behavior modification: II. Judgements and inferences of the clinician. *Cognitive Therapy and Research, 9,* 19-34.

Vallis, T. M., Shaw, B. F., & Dobson, K. S. (1986). The cognitive therapy scale: Psychometric properties. *Journal of Consulting and Clinical Psychology, 54,* 381-385.

Vallis, T. M., Shaw, B., & McCabe, S. (1988). The relationship between therapist competency in cognitive therapy and general therapy skill. *Journal of Cognitive Psychotherapy: An International Quarterly, 2,* 237-250.

Williams, J., & Spitzer, R. (Eds.). (1984). *Psychotherapy research: Where are we and where should we go?* New York: Guilford.

Wolpe, T. (1969). *The practice of behavior therapy.* New York: Pergamon Press.

Young, J. E., & Beck, A. T. (1980). *Cognitive therapy scale: Rating manual.* Unpublished manuscript. Center for Cognitive Therapy, Philadelphia, PA.

Young, J. E., & Beck, A. T. (1982). Cognitive therapy: Clinical applications. In A. J. Rush (Ed.), *Short-term psychotherapies for depression* (pp. 182-214). New York: Guilford.

Zajonc, R. (1984). On the primacy of affect. *American Psychologist, 39,* 151-175.

# 2

# Conceptualization and Flexibility in Cognitive Therapy

## Janice L. Howes and Carol A. Parrott

## Overview

Conceptualization in psychotherapy refers to the process of formulating and understanding a patient's problems within a specific framework. In cognitive therapy, the conceptualization of a patient's problems is a necessary aspect of therapy and an activity that usually precedes the implementation of specific therapeutic techniques. Much work has gone into developing cognitive conceptual frameworks to understand depression and anxiety. The view of depression as involving the perception of loss, and anxiety as involving the perception of threat, has been widely accepted. These general conceptual frameworks have been influential and useful in advancing the application and evaluation of cognitive therapy (Beck & Emery, 1985; Beck, Rush, Shaw, & Emery, 1979). It is equally important, however, in clinical work, to develop an idiosyncratic conceptualization which takes into account the patient's own development and personal history, resources, and environment (Beck *et al.*, 1979). From the extensive work that has been devoted to cognitive therapy, a number of frameworks have been developed from which to conceptualize a patient's problems. Therapists are now faced with choices about which cognitive conceptualization to follow in a given case.

The purpose of this chapter is to provide guidelines for developing

Janice L. Howes • Department of Psychiatry, Dalhousie University, and Department of Psychology, Camp Hill Medical Center, Halifax, Nova Scotia B3H 3G2, Canada. Carol A. Parrott • Private Practice, 1060 Springhill Drive, Mississauga, Ontario L5H 1M9, Canada.

idiosyncratic conceptualizations, particularly when working with non-traditional populations. We use the phrase traditional populations to refer to unipolar depression and anxiety disorders. In presenting these guidelines, we review the different conceptual frameworks currently available. These frameworks involve conceptualizations based on cognitive content, cognitive content versus cognitive process versus structure (labeled the tripartite conceptualization), core versus peripheral cognitive processes, constructivist and developmental processes, and finally, cognitive-interpersonal processes. The process of conceptualizing in cognitive therapy will be illustrated with a clinical example. The importance of flexibility in cognitive therapy with nontraditional patient groups will also be highlighted.

## CONTENT-BASED CONCEPTUALIZATION

One of the most unique and productive aspects of cognitive therapy is its focus on phenomenology. As such, the content of a patient's experience is perhaps the most obvious area of intervention. There is much empirical support for the efficacy of interventions targeted at cognitive content. Within cognitive therapy for anxiety and depressive disorders much of the therapeutic work is focused on cognitive content. A good example of this is a protocol-based approach to cognitive therapy, such as that employed in the National Institute of Mental Health Treatment of Depression Collaborative Research Program (TDCRP; Elkin, Parloff, Hadley, & Autry, 1985). Within this short-term protocol (usually 20 sessions), therapists focus primarily on education and symptom relief by directly assessing, and then intervening upon, the patient's automatic thoughts, beliefs, and expectations (cognitive content), using a variety of cognitive therapy-specific interventions (see Beck et al., 1979).

In cognitive therapy for *depression*, one of the major goals is to relieve emotional distress "by focusing on the patient's misinterpretations, self-defeating behavior, and dysfunctional attitudes" (Beck et al., 1979, p. 35). The most important cognitive content component of this conceptualization of depression is the negative cognitive triad. The negative cognitive triad involves a negative view of the self, a negative view of one's experiences, and a negative view of the future. It is important to note that the negative cognitive triad is not the only component of Beck's cognitive model of depression. In addition to the negative cognitive triad, important emphasis is placed on faulty information-processing styles and dysfunctional schemata (see next section). Nonetheless, one way of conceptualizing a patient's problem in cognitive therapy is to identify the unique content characteristics displayed by individuals with specific disorders. It is likely true that the majority of cognitive therapy-specific interventions are targeted at the level of cognitive content.

In terms of a content-focused conceptualization of *anxiety* disorders, Beck and Emery (1985) emphasize the cognitive concepts of danger and vulnerability. Beck proposes that anxiety-disordered individuals display a problem in the regulatory function of their cognitive system and that this leads to interpreting many environmental events as "dangers." Appraisal of danger produces a generalized sense of vulnerability. Automatic thoughts are generally conditional in anxiety disorders, as opposed to absolute and unconditional as in depression (e.g., "If X happens, something bad will happen to me"). Other examples of therapies that rely heavily on cognitive content include Meichenbaum's self-instructional training (1977) and Ellis's rational-emotive therapy (e.g., Ellis & Greiger, 1977).

Conceptualizing a patient's problem at a cognitive content level has a number of advantages. Immediate material that influences affect and behavior can be identified in a manner that the patient can easily relate to. Also, content-based conceptualizations lend themselves well to adaptation to nontraditional populations because they are largely descriptive. Thus, the therapist can construct an idiosyncratic model of a patient's phenomenology by focusing on problem issues (i.e., affect and behaviors) and probing retrospecitvely, prospectively, and immediately for cognitions, using available cognitive therapy tools (such as imagery rehearsal, role play, thought records). The chapters in Part II of this text illustrate the relevance of such content-based conceptualizations.

Despite these advantages, content-based conceptualizations are limited. Perhaps the major limitation is that these conceptualizations do not address nonaccessible cognitive processes or structures. There is considerable research, both from the areas of cognitive psychology (e.g., Craik and Tulving's [1975] depth of processing model) and cognitive therapy (e.g., Goldfried, Padawer, & Robins, 1984), indicating that nonaccessible cognitive processes play a role in emotional and behavioral disorders. A second limitation applies to the well-established models of depression and anxiety. Specifically, therapists must be cautious not to apply the models too rigorously. Not all depressed patients necessarily have all features of the negative cognitive triad. Individual differences must be taken into account in clinical work. As well, therapists must work to develop content-based conceptualizations for different disorders and not apply existing models (e.g., for depression) to contexts in which the model may be inappropriate (e.g., with personality disorders).

## TRIPARTITE CONCEPTUALIZATION

The tripartite conceptualization developed from increased interest in the role of information processing in psychopathology and in patient change in cognitive therapy (Hollon & Kriss, 1984). Beck *et al.* (1979) distinguish between automatic thoughts, faulty information-processing styles, and dysfunctional assumptions, and Hollon and Kriss (1984) differentiate cognitive factors into products, structures, and processes. This type of tripartite conceptualization (i.e., content, structures, and processes) advances our understanding of patients' problems beyond a content-based approach to a more dynamic approach, in that cognitive content, structures, and processes interact, and interventions at any level may be appropriate.

In this tripartite conceptualization, *cognitive products* (or content) consist of informational content and are the output of information processing. In cognitive therapy, cognitive products are generally referred to as self-statements by Meichenbaum (1977), automatic thoughts by Beck and his colleagues (1979), and beliefs by Ellis and Greiger (1977).

*Schemata* (or structures) are regarded as cognitive structures that contain specific information about situations and general information in the form of rules or "prototypic information" (Turk & Salovey, 1985a). Schemata serve a storage function for old information and play a role in the processing of new information. Self-schemata (i.e., information about the self and views of the self) are particularly important in clinical work. Cognitive psychology paradigms (e.g., incidential recall, Stroop Color-Naming Task) have been used to validate the operation of self-schemata in emotional disorders (e.g., Kuiper & Derry, 1982; Segal, Hood, Shaw, & Higgins, 1988). Clinically, much attention is placed on identifying the information composing the patient's self-schemata related to problem issues.

Cognitive *processes*, on the other hand, are viewed as the means by which deep cognitive structures are transformed into surface structures, and how existing information is recalled and existing cognitive structures activated or changed (Hollon & Kriss, 1984). Cognitive processes are often viewed as responsible for maladaptive cognitive content (i.e., thoughts) and the rigid quality of specific cognitive schemata. Several shortcomings in cognitive processing, such as selective attention, schema-confirming biases, egocentric biases, and illusory correlation, can contribute to patient problems (Turk & Salovey, 1985a, 1985b). Therapists may also display biases in cognitive processes that may adversely impact on the conceptualization of the patient and his/her problems. For example, if a patient has already been prelabeled as displaying borderline or antisocial personality features at the time of referral, this can influence the therapist's conceptualization and may result in confirmatory bias.

Beck's cognitive therapy (Beck *et al.*, 1979; Beck & Emery, 1985) is based on this tripartite model. For instance, with depression, Beck advocates three major concepts: the negative cognitive triad (content or products, to use Hollon & Kriss's 1984 terminology), cognitive errors or faulty information processing (processes), and dysfunctional assumptions (schemata or structures). The negative cognitive triad was explained in the previous section. As the patient becomes more depressed, his/her thinking becomes dominated by self-defeating assumptions (e.g., "unless I am successful at everything I try, I am worthless"). Various cognitive errors (distortions) in the thinking of the depressed patient add strength to his/her negative assumptions (e.g., arbitrary inference, selective abstraction, overgeneralization, magnification, minimization, and dichotomous thinking). Beck and Emery (1985) adopt a similar approach with anxiety disorders. As mentioned earlier, content focuses on danger and vulnerability. Cognitive distortions and dysfunctional assumptions operate much the same as with depression.

This tripartite conceptualization of patient difficulties in cognitive therapy allows us to look beyond cognitive content and begin to identify deeper-level cognitive factors. Interventions focused directly on process and structure often become central to progress in therapy. Despite the advantages of attending to cognitive processes and schemata, tripartite conceptualizations are limited in that they do not guide the therapist in deciding which are the most important cognitive factors to intervene on. As well, the patient's developmental and interpersonal history may be overlooked.

## CORE CONCEPTUALIZATION

Attention to cognitive structures, and more specifically self-schemata, has led some cognitive therapists to differentiate between surface- and deeper-level cognitions. Kelly (1955) was one of the first theorists to note levels of cognitive structures and also to differentiate core constructs (i.e., those governing "a person's maintenance processes," p. 482) from peripheral constructs (i.e., those which can be changed without alteration of core structures). In Kelly's personal construct theory, cognitive structures were hierarchically organized.

More recently, Safran, Vallis, Segal, and Shaw (1986) proposed that not all negative or upsetting thoughts have equal salience and importance. Some thoughts were viewed as being more central to the patient's problems than others. Based on Kelly's work, Safran et al. distinguished core and peripheral cognitive structures. According to Safran et al., core cognitive structures "are related to the definition and experience of the self" (p. 512). They are tacit in nature and are not easily accessed. Core cognitions can be used to predict a patient's emotional and behavioral responses in a variety of situations. Attempts to change core or central beliefs are assumed to result in greater anxiety, but to lead to longer-lasting change. Peripheral cognitions, on the other hand, are not derived from core cognitive structures and do not relate directly to the concept of self. They are explicit in nature and are more accessible than core structures. Changes in peripheral cognitions are assumed to evoke less anxiety and result in shorter-term change (Guidano & Liotti, 1983; Safran et al., 1986).

A brief case example illustrates the difference between core and peripheral cognitions. Consider a socially anxious patient who reported the following automatic thoughts: "I am going to make a fool of myself," "People are going to laugh at me," and "I can't do it." These automatic thoughts may derive from beliefs such as "I am an inadequate person" or "My value depends on what others think of me." One can see how the above automatic thoughts may derive from these beliefs about the self. These beliefs, if strongly involved in the patient's view of himself/herself, and if an integral aspect of his/her distress, would be conceptualized as being core. Beliefs such as "I would like to be successful" or "It is awful when things don't work out fairly" would be seen as peripheral beliefs, if they are not heavily involved in the patient's view of himself/herself.

Although conceptualizing at the level of core and peripheral cognitive structures appears to be clinically useful (Safran et al., 1986), there is very little empirical research addressing the core versus peripheral distinction. However, research employing the self-reference paradigm in controlled-processing studies provides some support for the notion that performance (i.e., memory) is superior under self-referent conditions due to the integration of the to-be-processed information into a structure of self-related concepts (Rogers, Kuiper, & Kirker, 1977). It should be noted that this paradigm has recently been criticized (e.g., Higgins & Bargh, 1987; Segal, 1990) for several shortcomings (e.g., failure to obtain better performance for words rated as self-descriptive relative to those rated as non-self-descriptive, inconsistency of predictions related to response latency).

Automatic-processing tasks such as the Stroop Color-Naming Task have been viewed by some researchers as an alternative to controlled-processing studies (Higgins & Bargh, 1987; Segal, Hood, Shaw, & Higgins, 1988). Some of these studies support the idea that automatic processing of self-related stimuli results in greater cognitive interference than non-self-related information (Segal *et al.*, 1988; see Louisy, 1989), whereas others have reported mixed findings. Few researchers have employed idiographic measures.

In a recent study, Louisy, Genest, Amsel, and Cheesman (1989; Louisy, 1989) attempted to operationalize and distinguish core versus peripheral beliefs. They developed a questionnaire to generate, and then categorize, idiographic self-descriptive trait adjectives. They then employed this approach to compare the cognitive interference associated with core trait adjectives and peripheral trait adjectives in a Stroop task. Words were classified as core trait adjectives based on accessibility (i.e., they were easily generated and assumed to be used by subjects to describe themselves generally) and cross-situational consistency (i.e, they were context-independent self-descriptive adjectives). Peripheral trait adjectives were identified by exclusion criteria. Louisy *et al.* found support for the validity of the core and peripheral distinction, as well as partial support for a distinction between the automatic processing of core and peripheral self-knowledge or beliefs (i.e., core trait adjectives resulted in significantly longer response latencies than peripheral adjectives). While more research is clearly needed in this area, these results, in conjunction with the self-reference paradigm findings, support the idea of cognitive schemata about the self, as well as offer empirical support for the clinical distinction of core and peripheral self-knowledge.

In order to *access core cognitive structures* clinically, the therapist attends to the patient's automatic thoughts and looks for patterns. The therapist must actively construct hypotheses based on the accessible cognitions, then test these hypotheses, altering them as needed when confronted with confirmatory or disconfirmatory evidence. This approach to conceptualization can be difficult for novice therapists, who may overattend to interventions to facilitate rapid change, and overlook the importance of core cognitive processes as they relate to enduring change (Safran *et al.*, 1986).

As outlined by Safran *et al.* (1986), there are several strategies one can employ to guide the conceptualization of core versus peripheral cognitions. First, vertical exploration can be employed. Safran *et al.* distinguish vertical from horizontal exploration. *Horizontal exploration* refers to the process of examining several automatic thoughts or peripheral cognitions without attending to the degree of centrality to the self. *Vertical exploration*, on the other hand, involves examining cognitions with respect to the meaning vis-à-vis the self. In vertical exploration, a frequently used and helpful question is "What does this mean about you as a person?" (see Safran *et al.*, 1986). A similar strategy has been described by Burns (1980) and by DeRubeis and Beck (1988) as the "downward arrow technique."

Other strategies to distinguish core from peripheral cognitions involve identifying common themes in cognitions (such as achievement or affiliation) and constancy across situations that produce symptoms or distress (e.g., conflict situations, isolation). Additionally, it has been hypothesized that core or central cognitions are more available to awareness in affectively charged states (Safran *et al.*, 1986). Beck *et al.* (1979) also emphasized the importance of attending to mood and affective shifts in therapy, since these can provide information about important cognitions. Thus, affect can be regarded as a process marker. For example, a patient with posttraumatic stress disorder who becomes very distraught when he states "I seem to be frightened of everything now" may be reflecting the core belief of generalized vulnerability (see Chapter 5, this volume).

Another opportunity for the therapist to obtain information concerning core cognitive structures occurs when treatment strategies fail. If core cognitions are generally more resistant to change than peripheral cognitions, failed interventions may serve as an opportunity to identify core cognitions. Probing for meaning vis-à-vis the self is highly recommended at this time. In a sense, resistance becomes a constructive process in terms of identifying core cognitions (akin to the "protective belt" identified by Guidano & Liotti, 1983; see also Chapter 3, this volume).

Conceptualizing patient problems in terms of core versus peripheral cognitions can facilitate treatment by identifying those cognitive structures most likely to produce lasting change. This approach also allows for greater understanding of patient problems by attempting to identify core beliefs, which may serve an organizing function for the individual. Finally, this approach may be useful in guiding treatment with more difficult patient populations, given its idiosyncratic focus. Despite these strengths, this approach has several disadvantages. First, it is time-consuming to access core cognitive structures and may not be suitable in some therapy situations. Second, core beliefs are hypothetical constructs and, thus, are always tentative. Finally, given the current lack of empirical verification for this approach, the reliability of such a distinction may be questionable.

## DEVELOPMENTAL-CONSTRUCTIVIST CONCEPTUALIZATION

As noted above, Guidano and Liotti (1983; Guidano, 1988) have also differentiated deep (tacit) and surface (explicit) cognitive structures.

However, they place their work within a developmental, constructivist perspective (see Chapter 1, this volume). They regard therapy as "an exploratory collaboration enabling the client to identify the basic assumptions underlying his or her way of experiencing reality" (pp. 326-327, Guidano, 1988). The therapist works to reconstruct the tacit rules underlying the patient's maladaptive behavior, and then facilitates the assimilation of new events and past memories into the patient's tacit knowledge of self.

According to Guidano and Liotti (1983), deep structures often have a developmental basis. That is, early developmental events often contribute to deep cognitive structures. Therefore, it is important to focus on the patient's cognitive, as well as emotional, development. Guidano and Liotti (1983) recommend that a careful developmental history be taken to help the therapist identify and access deep (core) cognitive structures in order to advance conceptualization. Guidano's (1988) conceptualization of agoraphobia is helpful in illustrating the impact of early developmental history. Guidano notes that some agoraphobics develop a belief that the world is not safe. This can often be associated with overprotective parents who limited the child's exploratory behavior and autonomy. As the agoraphobic grows older, he/she often develops an "outward, overly controlling attitude toward interpersonal relationships in order to obtain protection," as well as an "inward overly controlling attitude" toward his/her own perceived weakness (p. 335). Thus, he/she begins to fear any loss of control due to these underlying beliefs. Thoughts pertaining to loss of control then create anxiety (Guidano, 1988).

In addition to content, tripartite, and core versus peripheral frame works from which to conceptualize in cognitive therapy, a developmental conceptualization can also be added. The important question then becomes, under what conditions does such a conceptual model add to the previous frameworks. We contend that when clinical interventions based on previous frameworks fail, or when dealing with certain populations (e.g., personality disorders), it is useful to alter one's conceptual framework to include developmental issues.

## INTERPERSONAL-BASED CONCEPTUALIZATION

Another recent development focuses on the integration of cognitive and interpersonal approaches to therapy (e.g., Safran, 1984; Safran & Greenberg, 1988). This development has clear implications for the conceptualization of patient problems, as well as for treatment. Safran (1984; Safran & Segal, 1990) highlights the value of Sullivan's (1953) interpersonal theory to cognitive therapy and emphasizes the importance of the "cognitive-interpersonal cycle." Specifically, Safran states that cognitive, interpersonal, and interactional (i.e., "me-you patterns") factors are linked together in a cycle and that information processing in the real world involves "hot cognitions" (i.e., emotionally laden cognitions; see Safran & Greenberg, 1982, 1986). Safran proposes that the assessment of any single element of this cycle will affect the assessment of the others. One of the central points Safran makes is that the therapist can use the therapeutic context and relationship to generate information about the patient's core cognitions and problematic relationships, as well as use the relationship to intervene.

Jacobson (1989) also advocates the active use of the therapeutic relationship as a means to evaluate, test, and help the patient change core beliefs. Incorporating interpersonal factors into the cognitive conceptualization tends to result in greater attention being paid to the patient's cognitions, behaviors, and affect during the therapy session, as well as the therapist's feelings and responses that the patient evokes (Jacobson, 1989). In this way, the therapeutic relationship can be helpful in identifying core cognitions and can also become a training ground for developing healthier interpersonal relationships. An interpersonal-based conceptualization implies that the therapist may focus more specifically on the "here and now," may employ more Gestalt techniques to help deal with "hot cognitions," and may utilize behavioral strategies such as modeling and role playing within the context of the relationship, in addition to more standard cognitive techniques (see Safran & Segal, 1990).

## Guidelines to Conceptualization in Cognitive Therapy

All cognitive therapists would agree that the conceptualization of a patient's problem is necessary prior to implementing specific therapeutic techniques. As indicated by the above review, there are currently a number of conceptual frameworks available to the cognitive therapist. The availability of multiple frameworks allows one to approach conceptualization in a flexible manner, choosing the framework that best applies to the patient's individual difficulties. As the following case illustrates, limited attention to core cognitions, interpersonal variables, and developmental issues during conceptualization can result in difficulties during the intervention phase. For example, treating an agoraphobic patient with relaxation training can be problematic, or counterproductive, if control is a central, developmentally relevant issue for the patient, and if relaxation techniques are viewed as a threat to personal control by the patient (Liotti, 1984; Guidano, 1988). In this situation, attention to and delineation of the central issue of control would facilitate treatment by guiding the selection of the most appropriate treatment strategies. If relaxation is considered an important intervention in such a case, active forms of relaxation (e.g., self-directed imagery, walking) may be more appropriate.

Given the number of available conceptual models within cognitive therapy, the issue of which framework is most appropriate in which situation becomes central. The following guidelines, while not based on empirical research, can be helpful in the process of choosing an appropriate cognitive conceptual framework in clinical practice. We recommend a hierarchical approach to conceptualization. Movement from one level to the next is based on the patient's progress, his/her response to therapeutic strategies, and intervention targets. It is noteworthy that movement from one level to the next is not always sequential and consecutive.

We suggest the therapist begin by conceptualizing the problems at the cognitive content level. Cognitive content is most directly accessible. Further, there exists a wide range of specific cognitive therapy strategies directed at changing the content of cognitions. When such strategies fail, or when the patient has apparently gained as much as he/she can from content-focused interventions, the therapist should move to the tripartite conceptual framework. Here the therapist differentiates among cognitive content, cognitive structure, and cognitive process, and uses this information to obtain a clearer conceptualization of the patient's problem. This level of analysis elicits a deeper understanding of the patient's difficulties and the relevance of the difficulties to the self-schemata. Generally, this approach is more time-consuming.

In some cases, the tripartite level of analysis may be sufficent to understand and help resolve the problems, but if it is not, we recommend that the therapist differentiate cognitive structure according to core and peripheral beliefs (i.e., the core-peripheral conceptual framework). As illustrated above, this level of conceptualization requires a range of techniques to access core beliefs. Generally, this level of conceptualization occurs later in therapy, because of the inaccessibility of core beliefs and the need to accumulate relevant information prior to hypothesizing about core beliefs. Also, it is important to select out patients who respond to more straightforward and less time-consuming interventions. Once the therapeutic value of this framework has been exhausted, we recommend that the therapist incorporate a developmental analysis of the patient's problems, as suggested by Guidano and Liotti. It is helpful to explore how the patient's developmental, emotional, and cognitive history affected his/her current problems and may affect the outcome of treatment. Finally, we recommend that the ongoing process of conceptualization be conducted within the interpersonal context of the therapeutic relationship. That is, the importance of the therapeutic relationship as a means of assessment and intervention should be considered throughout therapy. It is also important to recognize the role of interpersonal factors in the patient's problems. We offer these suggestions as general guidelines. Therapists must approach conceptualization in a flexible manner, since some frameworks may be more appropriate with some populations than others (e.g., depression versus personality disorders).

## Case Example

A clinical case will be presented to illustrate this hierarchical approach to conceptualization. This case is one in which all levels of cognitive conceptualization were helpful in understanding the patient's presenting problem and in developing intervention strategies. As stated earlier, it may not be necessary for the clinician to explore or adopt all levels of conceptualization in individual cases. The transition from one level to another is determined on the basis of patient progress and intervention targets. As noted above, this process is not always sequential.

K.P. was a 36-year-old woman who worked as a secretary. She had a 10-year history of bipolar affective disorder with dependent personality features. She had been fairly well controlled with psychiatric support and medication (i.e., lithium carbonate). Over the years, she was hospitalized briefly on two occasions for depression following manic episodes. It is noteworthy that she had had only two brief manic episodes, but had felt depressed most of her life. She was referred for cognitive therapy following her last hospitalization.

At the time of initial assessment, she presented as clinically depressed, but denied severe depression. She reported feeling stressed and anxious, but was eager to improve and return to work. She was frequently troubled by racing thoughts, ruminations, and palpitations. She viewed herself in a negative manner. She reported a history of concern about her weight and having never felt positive about herself in the past. She was also having difficulty saying no to family members (especially her son and father), because she was fearful "something bad" would happen to them.

Her Millon Clinical Multiaxial Inventory (Millon, 1983) profile revealed the prominence of anxiety, dysthymic, and dependent features, and her Beck Depression Inventory (Beck, 1987) score revealed moderate depression. K.P. reported a longstanding problematic relationship with her father. Her mother, to whom she was close, died when K.P. was 14. K.P. completed high school and then a Bachelor of Nursing degree. However, she chose not to work as a nurse because she was uncertain of her abilities. She described a good work history as a secretary. She and her husband divorced following 10 years of marriage, and she had not seen him for 4 years. Her relationship with her 13-year-old son was fairly good, but at times she had difficulty managing his behavior.

Conceptualizing this patient's problems at a content level highlights K.P.'s negative view of herself, her abilities, and the future (i.e., the standard negative cognitive triad). Detailed inquiry and prospective thought monitoring produced the following characteristic automatic thoughts:

"I am a fat, unpleasant person."

"I am unable to say no to others."

"I cannot function at home."

"If my employer finds out I have an emotional disorder, he will fire me."

"This form of treatment is my last chance."

The therapeutic strategies appropriate to deal with problems at this conceptual level include coping self-thoughts and basic cognitive restructuring focusing on her negative view of herself, her abilities, and the future. In this case, however, an early attempt by the therapist to help the patient alter these dysfunctional thoughts was of limited benefit. Specifically, the patient had difficulty employing coping strategies and did not believe she could change dysfunctional thoughts with such strategies (e.g., coping self-statements, testing out negative thoughts). This suggested to the therapist that it was time to more fully explore her cognitions and to try to identify deeper-level cognitions.

Further exploration of K.P.'s cognitions and view of herself resulted in the identification of more specific cognitions related to a schema of self. The following beliefs were identified:

"I cannot say no to others, because I may hurt someone."

"I am useless, except when I am working."

"I have no positive personal attributes."

"My work being has nothing to do with my personal being."

"I should not express my opinion because I am always wrong."

As illustrated by these beliefs, this patient had low self-esteem, compartmentalized her personal self from her work self (dichotomous thinking), and was unable to say no because she believed someone might be hurt. Given the nature of this patient's problem, the evolving understanding of her self-schema, and the limited success of initial content-focused interventions, the therapist began to focus on core cognitive issues. Vertical exploration (Safran *et al.*, 1986) revealed the following core beliefs:

'If I say no to someone, I believe I will cause something horrible to happen to them and they may die."

"If others find out I have emotional problems, they will view me as unstable, I will lose my job, and then I will be completely
    useless."

"My opinions and feelings are not important because I am useless and unworthy."

Identification and discussion of these core beliefs resulted in K.P. acknowledging their relevance, but it was difficult for her to decenter and to test out these beliefs in an attempt to alter them. To obtain a clearer conceptualization, the therapist focused on the patient's developmental history, especially in regard to emotional issues and how she viewed herself in the past.

> K.P. reported that her mother had told her that she was dying when K.P. was 14. Early in the day a few weeks later, her mother had requested that a physician be called. K. P. tried to call a physician, but did not because her father did not think it was necessary. The physician was called by her father later that same day, but her mother died soon after. The patient believed that she was responsible for her mother's death because she had not disobeyed her father and had not called the physician immediately. From that time on, she reported feeling depressed much of the time and viewed herself as being a failure. Although she completed her Bachelor of Nursing degree, she chose not to work in nursing, because she was fearful that she might let another person die. Throughout her marriage, her husband physically abused her. Similarly, her father had verbally abused her throughout her childhood and adulthood. Collectively, her belief that she had been responsible for her mother's death (whom she had loved), and that she had allowed her father and her husband to abuse her, led to her core belief of being useless and unworthy.

Based on this additional information, it appeared that since age 14, K.P. had blamed herself for an event which was out of her control, and since that time she had continued to evaluate all negative events as being her fault. At this point, a decentering strategy ("that was then, this is now") was useful in helping the patient gain a clearer understanding of her dysfunctional thoughts and behavior.

These developmental issues emphasized the importance of the interpersonal context to this patient's problems. Further exploration revealed that K.P. was fearful that in some way she might be responsible for causing future harm to her son, whom she also loved. This contributed to her tendency to act in an unassertive and submissive manner with him. Similarly, the fact that she had tolerated abuse from her father and husband fed into her core belief that she was unworthy of love and was useless. Due to the past history of verbal and physical abuse, she had difficulty trusting others.

The conceptualization of this patient's problems in terms of core beliefs within a developmental and interpersonal context evolved over several sessions. Although K.P. obtained some benefit from interventions directed at content- and tripartite-level conceptualizations, exploration of their limits led to the modification of the conceptual framework. Since trust was an issue for the patient, it was necessary to establish a strong therapeutic alliance. Genuineness and empathy on the part of the therapist were important, as well as objective feedback to K.P. regarding her behavior and coping strategies. K.P. was psychologically minded and introspective, and she was receptive to the evolving conceptualization of her problems. Cognitive restructuring and coping strategies (e.g., coping self-statements, distraction, relaxation, and role playing) again became a focus in therapy, but only after the full conceptual framework was articulated and the patient was prepared for these content-based interventions. Dysfunctional thought records provided useful information at this time.

As K.P. became more comfortable with content- and situational-based strategies, and as she began to feel more positive about herself, she was receptive to further challenges (i.e., decentering) and reappraisal of some of her core beliefs. The major core beliefs challenged concerned her responsibility for her mother's death and her view of herself as unworthy and useless. This latter belief was reappraised in regard to the inconsistency of this belief with her good work performance and the positive therapeutic alliance developed within therapy. In conclusion, if the therapist had adhered to a content-based conceptualization of K.P.'s problems, and had not explored deeper-level cognitions, progress would have been limited, and central aspects of K.P.'s core beliefs missed.

## FLEXIBILITY

Developments in conceptualization expand the therapist's armamentarium and facilitate a more sophisticated appreciation of the patient's suffering. In addition to being able to collect automatic thoughts and employ strategies to address them, the therapist is also able to examine what the automatic thoughts mean about the self. Thus, the focus expands from intervening at the level of automatic thoughts (content) to intervening at the level of core cognitive structures and processes that have developmental and interpersonal relevance. As discussed above, the developments in conceptualization highlight the need for a more flexible approach to conceptualization in cognitive therapy.

There is also a need for more flexibility in the process and structure of treatment. First, the length of treatment must be geared toward the patient's needs and his/her rate of progress, as well as reflect the therapist's conceptualization. Although the standard 20-session cognitive therapy protocol is sufficient for many patients, there are some patients (e.g., pain patients) for whom a lengthier treatment period would be advantageous (Jacobson, 1989). Second, the choice of therapeutic strategy should be based on the therapist's cognitive conceptualization, as well as his/her skill level with various therapeutic techniques. In a flexible cognitive therapy approach, the use of techniques from other therapeutic orientations, in addition to cognitive techniques, can be particularly useful (e.g., Gestalt techniques; see Arnkoff, 1981). Flexibility in technique selection also implies that specific therapeutic interventions may not be useful with specific patients due to underlying core beliefs and over-powering emotional distress (e.g., use of systematic desensitization in the treatment of traumatic phobias; see Chapter 5, this volume). Finally, the therapist must be sensitive to patient crises (suicide attempts and threats, withdrawal, anger) and respond in a flexible manner. This may mean putting aside specific issues being worked on for several sessions in order to help the patient deal with a crisis. These events often yield useful information about the patient and his/her problems. The importance of flexibility in conceptualization and treatment will be highlighted throughout Part II of this book.

## Conclusions

There are a number of conceptual models currently available to the cognitive therapist when conceptualizing a patient's problem. The availability of diverse models allows the therapist to approach conceptualization and treatment in a more flexible manner. This is particularly important when dealing with nontraditional patient groups (e.g., personality disorders, pain problems, posttraumatic stress disorders) for whom a content-based conceptual model may not be the most appropriate. We have suggested guidelines that the therapist can employ in the process of selecting a cognitive conceptual framework in individual cases. Basically, we propose a hierarchical model beginning with a content-based conceptualization and then focusing on tripartite and core conceptualizations and, finally, on developmental and interpersonal-based conceptualizations. Movement from one level of conceptualization to the next should be based on the patient's progress, response to therapeutic techniques, and intervention targets. Flexibility is not only important in conceptualization, but also in therapy process and structure.

There is little empirical work currently available comparing the usefulness of the various conceptual models in cognitive therapy. At the present time, future research is needed to determine under what circumstances, and for which patients and which problems, specific conceptual models apply best (see Dobson, 1988). As well, clinical and research work is needed to help therapists determine the most effective approaches to obtain information that can be used conceptually, especially with nontraditional patient groups.

# REFERENCES

Arnkoff, D. (1981). Flexibility in practicing cognitive therapy. In G. Emery, S. D. Hollon, & R. C. Bedrosian (Eds.), *New directions in cognitive therapy: A case book* (pp. 203-223). New York: Guilford.

Beck, A. T. (1987). *Beck Depression Inventory*. New York: The Psychological Corporation.

Beck, A. T., & Emery, G. (1985). *Anxiety disorders and phobias: A cognitive perspective*. New York: Basic Books.

Beck, A. T., Rush, A. J., Shaw, B. F., & Emery, G. (1979). *Cognitive therapy and depression*. New York: Guilford.

Burns, D. (1980). *Feeling good: The new mood therapy*. New York: New American Library.

Craik, F. I. M., & Tulving, E. (1975). Depth of processing and the retention of words in episodic memory. *Journal of Experimenal Psychology: General, 104,* 268-294.

DeRubeis, R. J., & Beck, A. T. (1988). Cognitive therapy. In K. S. Dobson (Ed.), *Handbook of cognitive-behavioral therapies* (pp. 273-306). New York: Guilford.

Dobson, K. (1988). The present and future of cognitive-behavioral therapies. In K. S. Dobson (Ed.), *Handbook of cognitive-behavioral therapies* (pp. 389-414). New York: Guilford.

Elkin, I., Parloff, M., Hadley, S., & Autry, J. (1985). NIMH treatment of depression collaborative research program: Background and research plan. *Archives of General Psychiatry, 42,* 305-316.

Ellis, A., & Greiger, R. (1977). *Handbook of rational-emotive therapy*. New York: Springer.

Goldfried, M., Padawer, N., & Robins, C. (1984). Social anxiety and the semantic structure of heterosocial interaction. *Journal of Abnormal Psychology, 93,* 87-97.

Guidano, V. F. (1988). A systems, process-oriented approach to cognitive therapy. In K. S. Dobson (Ed.), *Handbook of cognitive-behavioral therapies* (pp. 307-354). New York: Guilford.

Guidano, V. F., & Liotti, G. (1983). *Cognitive processes and emotional disorders: A structural approach to psychotherapy*. New York: Guilford.

Higgins, E. T., & Bargh, J. A. (1987). Social cognition and social perception. *Annual Review of Psychology, 38,* 369-425.

Hollon, S., & Kriss, M. (1984). Cognitive factors in clinical research and practice. *Clinical Psychology Review, 4,* 35-76.

Jacobson, N. S. (1989). The therapist-client relationship in cognitive behavior therapy: Implications for treating depression. *Journal of Cognitive Psychotherapy, 3,* 85-96.

Kelly, G. (1955). *The psychology of personal constructs.* New York: Norton.

Kuiper, N. A., & Derry, P. A. (1982). Depressed and nondepressed content self-reference in mild depressives. *Journal of Personality, 50,* 67-80.

Liotti, G. (1984). Cognitive therapy, attachment theory and psychiatric nosology. In M. A. Reda & M. J. Mahoney (Eds.), *Cognitive psychotherapies.* Cambridge, MA: Ballinger.

Louisy, H. (1989). *Automatic activation of core and peripheral self-knowledge: An idiographic approach.* Unpublished master's thesis, University of Saskatchewan, Saskatoon, Canada.

Louisy, H., Genest, M., Amsel, E., & Cheesman, J. (1989). *Automatic activation of core and peripheral self-knowledge: An idiographic approach.* Paper presented at Canadian Psychological Association Convention, Halifax, Nova Scotia.

Meichenbaum, D. (1977). *Cognitive behavior modification.* New York: Plenum.

Millon, T. (1983). Millon Clinical Multiaxial Inventory. Minneapolis, MN: Interpretive Scoring Systems.

Rogers, T. B., Kuiper, N. A., & Kirker, W. S. (1977). Self-reference and the encoding of personal information. *Journal of Personality and Social Psychology, 35*(9), 677-688.

Safran, J. D. (1984). Assessing the cognitive-interpersonal cycle. *Cognitive Therapy and Research, 8,* 333-348.

Safran, J. D., & Greenberg, L. S. (1982). Eliciting "hot cognitions" in cognitive behavior therapy: Rationale and procedural guidelines. *Canadian Psychologist, 23,* 83-87.

Safran, J. D., & Greenberg, L. S. (1986). Hot cognition and psychotherapy process: An information processing/ecological approach. In P. C. Kendall (Ed.), *Advances in cognitive-behavioral research and therapy* (pp. 143-177). New York: Academic Press.

Safran, J., & Greenberg, L. (1988). Feeling, thinking and acting: A cognitive framework for psychotherapy intergration. *Journal of Cognitive Psychotherapy: An International Quarterly, 2,* 109-131.

Safran, J., & Segal, Z. V. (1990). *Cognitive therapy: An interpersonal process perspective.* New York: Basic Books.

Safran, J., Vallis, T. M., Segal, Z. V, & Shaw, B. F. (1986). Assessment of core cognitive processes in cognitive therapy. *Cognitive Therapy and Research, 10,* 509-526.

Segal, Z. V. (1990). Appraisal of the self-schema construct in cognitive models of depression. *Psychological Bulletin, 103,* 147-162.

Segal, Z. V., Hood, J. E., Shaw, B. F., & Higgins, E. T. (1988). A structural analysis of the self-schema construct in major depression. *Cognitive Therapy and Research, 12,* 471-486.

Sullivan, H. S. (1953). *The interpersonal theory of psychiatry.* New York: Norton.

Turk, D., & Salovey, P. (1985a). Cognitive structures, cognitive processes, and cognitive behavior modification: I. Client issues. *Cognitive Therapy and Research, 9,* 1-18.

Turk, D., & Salovey, P. (1985b). Cognitive structures, cognitive processes, and cognitive behavior modification: II. Judgements and inferences of a clinician. *Cognitive Therapy and Research, 9,* 19-34.

# 3

# The Therapeutic Relationship and Resistance to Change in Cognitive Therapy

## MARSHA M. ROTHSTEIN AND PAUL J. ROBINSON

## INTRODUCTION

A positive therapeutic relationship is considered to be a necessary component of all forms of cognitive therapy, particularly as a necessary prerequisite for cognitive techniques to be effective (Beck, Rush, Shaw, & Emery, 1979; Guidano, 1987). However, the patient-therapist relationship can be seen as providing more than just the groundwork upon which cognitive-behavioral interventions occur (Guidano & Liotti, 1983; Safran & Segal, 1990). The therapeutic relationship itself can be used as an intervention to explore relevant issues in cognitive therapy. That is, the relationship can be the means to help certain patients identify, understand, and change cognitions and metacognitions which, in turn, may lead to more satisfying and enduring therapeutic change.

Resistance to change can occur even when a positive therapeutic relationship is established and maintained. There is a danger in cognitive therapy of viewing resistance as something to be minimized and overcome (Beck *et al.*, 1979; Dryden & Ellis, 1986; Meichenbaum & Gilmore, 1982) rather than as an adaptive and self-protective phenomenon (Mahoney, 1988). Indeed, resistance to change can be seen as a process marker (i.e., behavior that indicates an appropriate juncture for

MARSHA M. ROTHSTEIN • Independent Practice, Delisle Court Professional Center, 1560 Yonge Street, Suite 300, Toronto, Ontario M4T 2S9, Canada.    PAUL J. ROBINSON • Department of Psychology, North York General Hospital, Willowdale, Ontario M2K 1E1, Canada.

cognitive and emotional exploration; Safran & Segal, 1990), indicating to the therapist that an exploration of the patient's self- and interpersonal schemata may be needed. In our view, resistance to change is something to be respected and explored rather than eliminated.

In this chapter separate discussions of the therapeutic relationship, both as a prerequisite for technical interventions, and as an intervention itself, will be presented. As well, a proposal that links the therapeutic relationship and resistance to change will be presented.

## THE THERAPEUTIC RELATIONSHIP

### The Therapeutic Relationship as a Prerequisite for Technical Interventions

A review of the chronological development of contemporary cognitive-behavioral therapies (e.g., Dobson & Block, 1988) suggests that most cognitive therapists have endorsed Kelly's (1955) notion of the therapist and patient as "personal scientists" who observe, explore, and experiment with various aspects of the patient's world in a collaborative manner. Similar to Kelly's notion of personal scientists, Beck and colleagues (Beck et al., 1979) define collaborative empiricism as a team approach in which the patient supplies the raw data to be investigated with the therapist's guidance. It is clear that collaborative empiricism is fundamental to cognitive therapy. It has defined both explicitly and implicitly the objectives of a positive therapeutic relationship, the therapist characteristics needed to establish this relationship, and the process of cognitive therapy.

The *objective* of establishing a therapeutic relationship, as stated by Beck et al. (1979), is to "develop a milieu in which the specific cognitive change techniques can be applied most efficiently" (p. 46). Beck et al. discuss difficulties in the therapeutic relationship, such as "incapacitating transference," as technical problems. When these occur, the cognitions identified are examined in the same fashion as any other data (e.g., the evidence for the cognition is examined, alternative cognitions are considered, etc.). Nevertheless, Beck et al. advise cognitive therapists to minimize these types of problematic reactions in therapy. This perspective on dealing with problems arising in therapy is not unlike that taken by many other cognitive therapists, in which more attention is placed on technique and less on the relationship between the therapist and the patient (Meichenbaum, 1985; Rehm, 1977).

If the objective of the therapeutic relationship is to establish and maintain a therapeutic milieu that will promote successful technical interventions, then certain *therapist characteristics* are needed. Most cognitive therapists would agree that if the therapist demonstrates non-possessive warmth, accurate empathy, and genuineness, collaboration with the patient is enhanced (Beck *et al.*, 1979; Beck & Emery, 1985; D'Zurilla, 1988). Although these characteristics are not considered sufficient for cognitive and behavior changes to occur, they are considered necessary (Beck *et al.*, 1979).

In addition to possessing these characteristics, the therapist needs to function as an educator (Dobson & Block, 1988) who instructs, challenges, and reinforces the patient in his/her efforts to change dysfunctional beliefs and behaviors. Beck and Emery (1985) caution the therapist not to take a superior role in this process, but to develop the relationship on a reciprocal basis (the collaboration in collaborative empiricism). By being open and direct, by admitting mistakes, and by encouraging the patient's input and feedback, the therapist communicates to the patient that they are partners in this effort.

Finally, guided by the notion of collaborative empiricism, the *process* of therapy takes on a highly interactive quality. The therapist actively engages the patient in devising and experimenting with strategies for cognitive and behavioral change and the patient responds by reporting the results of these activities. Both patient and therapist are very active in the therapy sessions. Activity level can vary according to the therapist's conceptualization of what is needed to maintain the working alliance, but adjustment of activity level is not considered an intervention *per se* (Beck & Emery, 1985).

## The Therapeutic Relationship as an Intervention

Although the therapeutic relationship has been discussed by cognitive therapists, as argued above, it has usually been considered within the context of maximizing the effectiveness of technical interventions. For instance, Lambert (1983), in his review of the importance attributed to the therapist-patient relationship within different therapies, concludes that cognitive therapists barely mention the relationship and/or view it as an administrative task. However, this is beginning to change (Safran & Segal, 1990). Cognitive therapists have begun to acknowledge and explore the important role that the therapeutic relationship plays in cognitive therapy. Arnkoff (1981), for example, was one of the first cognitive therapists to discuss how she uses the therapeutic relationship as a tool to help her patients understand that their conceptualizations of their relationships with her may be very similar to the ways in which they construe their relationships outside of therapy. More recently, Jacobson (1989) suggests that the therapeutic relationship can become an active vehicle for producing change in depressed patients. In order to produce long-term change, Jacobson concludes that the therapist-patient relationship "must be incorporated into the conceptual underpinnings of treatment" (p. 94).

One of the more comprehensive discussions of the use of the therapeutic relationship as an intervention in cognitive therapy has been provided by Guidano and Liotti (1983; Guidano, 1987). Guidano and Liotti endorse a "constructivist" approach to cognitive therapy (see Chapter 1, this volume) and place paramount importance upon the role of the therapeutic relationship in cognitive therapy. Their definitions of the objective of the relationship, the therapist characteristics needed to establish the relationship, and the process of therapy, differ from those of Beck and his colleagues (Beck *et al.*, 1979).

According to Guidano and Liotti (1983), the *objective* of the therapeutic relationship is defined by their statement that "the [patient's] ability to recognize the personal value and meaning of the feelings emerging in the therapeutic relationship is the most significant achievement of the psychotherapist's job" (p. 120). Their approach involves less focus on technical interventions than other cognitive therapy approaches (Beck *et al.*, 1979; Meichenbaum, 1985). Guidano's and Liotti's focus on uncovering personal meaning through the therapeutic relationship arises from their hypothesis that this relationship reflects the patient's developmental history, particularly his/her attachment patterns (Bowlby, 1977). Dysfunctional attachment patterns, they suggest, can prevent the integration of self-knowledge, which in turn may lead to clinical disturbance (Guidano, 1987). As such, an exploration of the patient's developmental processes in therapy can lead to the patient's understanding of how current self-knowedge arose and that certain self-schemata may no longer be adaptive. In addition, this exploration provides information to the therapist about issues that may arise within the therapeutic relationship (e.g., issues of trust, dependency, and aggression).

If the objective of the above approach is to help the patient understand the meaning of the feelings emerging in the therapeutic relationship, then an important *therapist characteristic* is flexibility. In addition to warmth, empathy, and genuineness, the therapist needs to be able to adjust his/her approach, depending upon the issues that arise from the exploration of developmental processes. Mahoney and Gabriel (1987) maintain that in order for the patient to maximize knowledge gained through therapy, the therapist needs to provide a safe place for the patient to explore interactions with self and world. The therapist can do this by interacting with the patient on the basis of the patient's self-constructs. For example, if the patient's self-definition includes dependency on others, the therapist initially may choose not to raise this issue vis-à-vis the therapeutic relationship until the patient appears comfortable in the relationship. At the appropriate time, the therapist may discuss the patient's dependency on the therapist and then help the patient understand the meaning of the feelings that may arise from this discussion. New knowledge of self that may evolve from this interaction could be integrated into old self-schemata, and more adaptive self-constructs could result.

Finally, the *process* of therapy changes when using the therapeutic relationship as an intervention. In order to fully explore the personal meaning of the feelings aroused in the relationship, the therapist at times may become less directive. Rather than directly challenging old beliefs and actively urging patients to accept new ones, the therapist encourages patients to explicitly acknowledge previous knowledge of self and "its intense, contradictory paradoxes and pitfalls" (Guidano & Liotti, 1983, p. 120). In an effort to accomplish this, the therapist minimizes the frequency of direct interventions to alter the patient's cognitions. Take, for example, the case of a male patient with social phobia who reports, "Women ignore me." The therapist might intervene at this point by encouraging the patient to take an active role in controlling or altering this thought (e.g., "Where is the evidence for this belief?" or "Let's find ways of helping you interact more skillfully with women"). Such a process is characterized by encouraging the patient to challenge, disconfirm, and adopt a more functional perspective. However, the process would be different when the focus is on the personal meaning of the therapeutic relationship. A female therapist might say, "Do you feel ignored by me?" and "What does it mean for you to have women ignore you?" By exploring the meaning of the patient-therapist interaction the therapist could probe for important (core) self-knowledge. Probing with the above questions not uncommonly produces responses such as, "I am a loser"; "I am unlovable." The goal here is to identify existing self-knowledge, not to force *new* knowledge on the patient. To arrive at an understanding of tacit assumptions about themselves and their world, patients are guided to recognize their own personal truths and are not persuaded to adopt others' standards of reality (Guidano, 1987). To achieve this goal the therapeutic process at times becomes less direct and active. More time is spent talking about the therapeutic relationship and its meaning to the patient than is spent actively challenging the patient's cognitions.

This use of the therapeutic relationship in cognitive therapy is also highlighted by Safran and Segal (1990) in their comprehensive attempt to integrate cognitive and interpersonal approaches to psychotherapy. Safran and Segal argue that the technical focus in cognitive therapy can result in an overreliance on the application of techniques, without an understanding of the process that makes the techniques work. Similar to Guidano and Liotti, they believe that the therapeutic relationship plays a critical role in the process of change. They hypothesize that interpersonal schemata (i.e., the individual's generic representation of self-other interactions) predispose the patient to develop clinical problems. It is these interpersonal schemata that must be modified in therapy if change is to be achieved. Safran and Segal (1990) suggest that this can be accomplished by testing out the patient's expectations of the therapeutic relationship. Not only is the patient's subjective experience in therapy regarded as important, but the therapist's feelings and action tendencies are also important indicators that can pinpoint specific patient problems (Safran, 1984).

In summary, there has been a recent trend by some cognitive therapists to reevaluate the role played by the therapeutic relationship in cognitive therapy (Jacobson, 1989; Safran & Segal, 1990). Not only is a positive therapeutic relationship necessary for effective technical interventions, but the relationship itself becomes a powerful tool for facilitating change at the level of cognitive structure and content.

## RESISTANCE

In any therapeutic approach in which there is a strong emphasis on technique, failure to change is easily seen as a problem to be solved. Although Beck et al. (1979) do not employ the term *resistance*, they do acknowledge that patients' counterproductive ideas and behaviors can slow down therapy. Golden (1983), on the other hand, operationally defines resistance as a failure of patients to comply with therapeutic procedures. Golden and Dryden (1986) recommend that, when dealing with resistance, cognitive-behavior therapists take a problem-solving approach by using the same methods as they do for any other problem in therapy.

From a cognitive therapy perspective, problems in resistance may be due to several factors, including patient, therapist, and/or patient-therapist relationship variables (Beck et al., 1979; Ellis, 1983a, 1983b; Lazarus, 1987). An example is provided by Beck et al. (1979), in which lack of progress in therapy is attributed to the *patient*. In the case of a patient who is chronically late and/or misses appointments, Beck et al.

recommend that the therapist attempt to ascertain the reasons for this behavior, without sounding accusatory. Nevertheless, if these problems are chronically manifested by the patient, Beck *et al.* recommend that the patient be told that if he or she wants treatment to be successful, the rules of treatment have to be followed (pp. 315-316). Such a recommendation seems to reflect a perception of resistance in cognitive therapy as a problem to be overcome, and of the patient as being difficult. Similarly, Ellis (1983a, 1983b, 1985; Dryden & Ellis, 1986) has described several patient obstacles to therapeutic progress. These include the patient's failure to do homework, failure to use self-disputation consistently, or failure to accept responsibility for inappropriate emotions. In addition, Lazarus (1987; Lazarus & Fay, 1982) has outlined two patient variables involved in treatment impasses. These include extreme excesses or deficits in the patient's functioning and/or the patient's undervaluing treatment outcome. It should be noted, however, that while patient variables need to be explored, if resistance is conceptualized only as a patient-related problem, the therapist runs the risk of blaming the patient for treatment failure.

*Therapist-related* factors that may contribute to resistance include the misapplication or inflexible use of techniques, or a mistaken focus on secondary rather than central problems (Beck & Young, 1984; Lazarus, 1987; Weishaar & Beck, 1986). As well, Ellis notes the problems of therapists' skill deficits or the presence of unresolved therapist disturbance as contributing to resistance. Solutions to these difficulties rest with therapists improving their skills or searching for and disputing their own self-defeating beliefs (Dryden & Ellis, 1986).

In addition to patient and therapist factors, the *therapeutic relationship* may be involved in resistance to change. For example, Ellis and Lazarus (Dryden & Ellis, 1986; Lazarus, 1987) suggest that a poor patient-therapist match may contribute to a treatment impasse. Ellis also describes therapist-patient collusion as a possible obstacle to treatment progress. This may occur as a result of both the patient's and therapist's low tolerance of anxiety in the therapy. In a further discussion of patient-therapist factors, Beck and Young (1984) suggest that, if the therapist notices the patient's anger or dissatisfaction with the therapist, it is critical to share this observation with the patient. If the problem seems based on misinterpretation, the standard approach of data collection, alternative explanations, and questioning is used. Thus, rather than viewing the patient as being stubbornly resistant, the therapist sees this as an opportunity to collect valuable data for understanding the presenting problem.

To this point, the views outlined above indicate a general perception of resistance as problematic. As recently noted by Liotti (1987), however, there has not been much attention paid to the relationship between resistance to change and what we know about the development, maintenance, and organization of cognition. This seems surprising, in light of the fundamental concern in the cognitive therapies with cognitive activities and functioning.

In contrast to this lack of attention to the *cognitive aspects* of resistance, Meichenbaum and Gilmore (1982) have discussed the association between resistance and cognitive processes. Specifically, these authors refer to the analogy of the scientific model, noting that scientists and patients alike are constrained by their "paradigms," or their "tacit knowledge." The paradigms and behavior of scientists are as resistant to change as are the paradigms and behavior of patients. Meichenbaum and Gilmore also conclude that patient resistance may reflect "perspicacious wisdom and plain good judgement" (p. 154), if the efficacy of a proposed treatment is not clear to the patient. These authors propose that underlying every resistance are cognitions of the general form, "trying to change is only going to risk that very likely possibility of making everything much worse" (p. 152). Both of these notions (i.e., the constraint imposed by personal paradigms, and the possibility that a patient is showing good judgment in protecting himself/herself from inappropriate treatment) seem to anticipate recent conceptual and therapeutic developments in the cognitive-behavioral literature.

Neimeyer (1986), whose work is based on personal construct theory (Kelly, 1955), argues that when therapeutic impasses occur, the therapist should not assume that this is the result of a defensive, resistant process. Instead, it could be thought of as a shortcoming in the patient's existing construct system (Neimeyer, 1986). In other words, the construct system of that individual does not support the insights the therapist thinks the patient should be able to realize. When this is the case, anxiety and a sense of threat may be manifested by the patient.

According to Neimeyer (1986), a personal construct therapist is guided by the overall goal of providing ideal conditions in therapy for the development of new constructs. Thus, rather than "disputing" the validity or logic of a patient's cognitions when the patient may be in this anxious and/or threatened state, the therapist assists the patient to consider alternative views and behaviors and encourages active experimentation and role playing, both within and outside of therapy sessions. Padesky (1988) also emphasizes the importance of building new schemata when assisting those patients who appear treatment resistant.

Liotti (1987) addresses the meaning of resistance by providing a relatively comprehensive cognitive conceptualization of it. In contrast to

the psychoanalytic explanation of resistance as a defense against unconscious drives and repressed memories, Liotti (1987) argues that the manifestation of so-called resistance reflects patients' attempts to preserve
their meaning structures. Achievement and preservation of meaning is
thought to be a primary aim of human mental functioning. Old structures of meaning, therefore, naturally will be resistant to change because
of individuals' innate need to predict and attribute meaning, and because of the stability afforded by an established meaning structure.

Based on a constructivist perspective (Guidano & Liotti, 1983), Liotti
(1987) also argues that mental processes are ordered according to a hierarchy of levels of organization. The higher-order, core organizing principles (that are very much related to the sense of personal identity, and
provide coherence and consistency in one's life) are more resistant to
change than are lower-order, peripheral processes (that change in response to environmental contingencies). Thus, challenging these core,
deep structures typically will be experienced by patients as a frightening
assault on their identity, and the manifested resistance actually may
reflect self-protective processes. Fransella's (1989) research with stutterers supports this argument. It was found that those stutterers who
had a strong concept of themselves as stutterers improved the least with
treatment. As Bugental and Bugental (1984) argue, resistance arises
when important life structures are imperiled. For many patients, change
is "a fate worse than death" (p. 543). As these authors further note,
"resistance is not solely that which blocks the patient's full living, it also
is what makes possible the ways in which the patient does live life" (p.
543).

In summary, the issue of resistance has received increased attention
by cognitive therapists and theorists. Typically, cognitive therapists
have tended to take a problem-solving approach when faced with patient resistance (Golden & Dryden, 1986; Liotti, 1987). This seems to
reflect an assumption that resistance is a practical or "technical" problem
(a "thing"; Fransella, 1989) that needs to be overcome by the therapist by
the use of technical solutions. Moreover, as Mahoney (1988) recently has
argued, cognitive therapists have generally viewed resistance as the
antithesis of change, and although such a development in therapy may
provide valuable information, it is something to be minimized. Until
recently, cognitive therapists have tended to consider resistance as an
unexpected, unfortunate, and unwelcome phenomenon. Alternative
conceptualizations, however, portray resistance as a normal process in
therapy that provides an opportunity to explore valuable information
about the patient's fundamental cognitive processes. According to this
conceptualization, resistance in therapy is expected, since it is thought

to reflect natural and healthy self-protective processes that guard against changing too much, too quickly. In therapy, therefore, it is useful if therapists respect the adaptive quality of resistance and attempt to work "with" rather than "against" this process.

## Use of the Therapeutic Relationship When Resistance Occurs

We have discussed how resistance to change at times can occur due to the misuse of techniques, and that it can be managed by altering technique. We have also discussed that resistance to change can alternatively be understood in terms of a threat to core constructs. In this case, resistance is thought to be adaptive and self-protective in nature. We propose that resistance can occur for both reasons.

The first reason (i.e., a therapeutic impasse may occur because the techniques applied are not appropriate) suggests that a modification of the technical intervention is needed. For example, a patient with an anxiety disorder may resist progressive relaxation training (Barlow, 1988). In exploring the reasons for the resistance the therapist may discover that the exercise is seen by the patient as too time-consuming. By modifying the time requirements the therapist increases the likelihood that the patient will try the exercise and will find symptom relief.

The second reason for resistance (i.e., core constructs are involved) suggests that a modification of technical interventions will not solve the problem. Two cues can be identified that suggest to the therapist that core processes are present. First, technical interventions are not working. Second, during a therapeutic impasse the therapy session becomes emotionally charged (by the patient's expression of certain feelings and or behavior).

If core cognitions can be accessed by the evocation of the emotions to which they are associated (Guidano & Liotti, 1983; Safran & Segal, 1990), and if a therapeutic impasse often involves "hot cognitions" (Greenberg & Safran, 1984), then an opportunity to access core cognitions arises when resistance occurs. If a general meaning inquiry about the emotions evoked is not productive, in the attempt to access this core material, the therapist can choose to turn to the therapeutic relationship. For example, in a therapy situation in which a discussion of a particular topic gives rise initially to a patient's anger and eventual withdrawal (i.e., he/she becomes silent or responds very cooly), the therapist has three choices. The first choice is to continue probing, which may result in exacerbating the patient's resistance (sometimes exploration of the personal meaning associated with the patient's emotions will result in an increase in anger or withdrawal). The second choice is to change topics, which may increase the patient's responsiveness, but not increase the understanding of the emotions. It is at these times that the therapist can turn to the therapeutic relationship as a third option.

In turning to the therapeutic relationship the therapist can discuss the patient's feelings, the shift in the patient's feelings from intense anger to coldness, and also the therapist's own feelings about the process that has occurred. Questions such as "What was it that provoked your anger in our discussion?" and "What did it mean for you to become so angry?" are meant to help the patient come to some understanding of the meaning of the emotions. Core constructs are likely to emerge from this interchange (e.g., "When I am questioned I feel criticized and become angry" or "If I am angry, people [like you] will reject me"). In addition, if the therapist describes his/her own feelings, such as "When you withdrew I became frustrated and wanted to withdraw also," the interpersonal schema of the patient also becomes a focus. The integration of old and new knowledge of self and others is facilitated by the use of the therapeutic relationship in this way. From this perspective, rather than viewing resistance as a negative factor in therapy, the therapist can anticipate the positive gains that may result when resistance is encountered.

## SUMMARY

In this chapter, we have provided an overview of the role played by the therapeutic relationship, and of the conceptualization of resistance, in cognitive therapy. As cognitive therapy has evolved over the past two decades the therapeutic relationship and resistance to change have received increased attention by cognitive therapists. Although work on these two aspects of therapy have developed somewhat separately in the cognitive therapy literature, it is our view that there is good reason to consider them conjointly. Resistance can occur under many circumstances, but the following two mechanisms should be highlighted: resistance that occurs when technical interventions are inappropriately applied, and resistance that occurs when core constructs are challenged. It is during the latter occurrence that the therapeutic relationship can be used as a powerful intervention. We concur with Safran and Segal (1990) that a good therapeutic relationship can be a *mechanism* of change, not simply a necessary condition for change. When the patient experiences a threat to his/her knowledge of self and others, and resists changing these dysfunctional core constructs, the therapeutic relationship can be the means to effect the necessary change. This perspective has implications for therapy objectives, therapist characteristics, and the process of therapy. One of the primary developments in cognitive therapy in the past five years has been an emphasis on process in therapy. This perspective implies that reseach methodology that addresses process issues in cognitive therapy (e.g., Greenberg & Safran, 1987) will become increasingly important, if the theoretical and clinical hypotheses we have discussed are to be empirically validated.

# References

Arnkoff, B. (1981). Flexibility in practicing cognitive therapy. In G. Emery, S. Hollon & R. Bedrosian (Eds.), *New directions in cognitive therapy* (pp. 203-223). New York: Guilford.

Barlow, D. H. (1988). *Psychological treatment of panic.* New York: Guilford.

Beck, A. T., & Emery, G. (1985) *Anxiety disorders and phobias.* New York: Basic Books.

Beck, A. T., & Young, J. (1984). Cognitive therapy of depression. In D. Barlow (Ed.), *Clinical handbook of psychological disorders: A step-by-step treatment manual* (pp. 204-206). New York: Guilford.

Beck, A. T., Rush, A. J., Shaw, B., & Emery, G. (1979). *Cognitive therapy of depression.* New York: Guilford.

Bowlby, J. (1977). The making and breaking of affectional bonds. *British Journal of Psychiatry, 130,* 421-431.

Bugental, J., & Bugental, E. (1984). A fate worse than death: The fear of changing. *Psychotherapy, 21,* 543-549.

Dobson, K. S., & Block, L. (1988). Historical and philosophical bases of the cognitive-behavioral therapies. In K. S. Dobson (Ed.), *Handbook of cognitive-behavioral therapies* (pp. 3-38). New York: Guilford.

Dryden, W., & Ellis, A. (1986). Rational-emotive therapy (RET). In W. Dryden & W. Golden (Eds.), *Cognitive-behavioral approaches to psychotherapy* (pp. 129-168). New York: Harper & Row.

D'Zurilla, T. J. (1988). Problem-solving therapies. In K. S. Dobson (Ed.), *Handbook of cognitive-behavioral therapies* (pp. 85-135). New York: Guilford.

Ellis, A. (1983a). Rational-emotive therapy (RET) approaches to overcoming resistance I: Common forms of resistance. *British Journal of Cognitive Therapy, 1,* 28-38.

Ellis, A. (1983b). Rational-emotive therapy (RET) approaches to overcoming resistance II: How RET disputes clients irrational resistance-creating beliefs. *British Journal of Cognitive Therapy, 1,* 1-16.

Ellis, A. (1985). *Overcoming resistance.* New York: Springer.

Fransella, F. (1989). Obstacles to change and the reconstruction process: A personal construct view. In W. Dryden & P. Trower (Eds.), *Cognitive psychotherapy: Stasis and change* (pp. 14-27). New York: Springer.

Golden, W. (1983). Resistance in cognitive-behavior therapy. *British Journal of Cognitive Psychotherapy, 1*(II), 33-42.

Golden, W., & Dryden, W. (1986) Cognitive-behavioral therapies: Commonalities, divergences, and future developments. In W. Dryden & W. Golden (Eds.), *Cognitive-behavioral approaches to psychotherapy* (pp. 356-378). New York: Harper & Row.

Greenberg, L. A., & Safran, J. D. (1984). Integrating affect and cognition: A perspective on therapeutic change. *Cognitive Therapy and Research, 8*, 559-578.

Greenberg, L. A., & Safran, J. D. (1987). *Emotion in psychotherapy: Affect, cognition and the process of change*. New York: Guilford.

Guidano, V. (1987). *Complexity of the self*. New York: Guilford.

Guidano, V., & Liotti, G. (1983). *Cognitive processes and emotional disorders*. New York: Guilford.

Jacobson, N. (1989). The therapist-client relationship in cognitive therapy implications for treating depression. *Journal of Cognitive Psychotherapy: An International Quarterly, 3*, 85-96.

Kelly, G. A. (1955). *The psychology of personal constructs*. New York: Norton.

Lambert, M. J. (1983). *Psychotherapy and patient relationships*. Homewood, IL: Dorsey.

Lazarus, A. (1987). The multimodal approach with adult outpatients. In N. Jacobson (Ed.), *Psychotherapists in clinical practice: Cognitive and behavioral perspectives* (pp. 286-326). New York: Guilford.

Lazarus, A., & Fay, A. (1982). Resistance or rationalization? A cognitive-behavioral perspective. In P. Wachtel (Ed.), *Resistance: Psychodynamic and behavioral approaches* (pp. 115-132). New York: Plenum.

Liotti, G. (1987). The resistance to change of cognitive structures: A counterproposal to psychoanalytic metapsychology. *Journal of Cognitive Psychotherapy: An International Quarterly, 1*, 87-104.

Mahoney, M. (1988). The cognitive sciences and psychotherapy: Patterns in a developing relationship. In K. Dobson (Ed.), *Handbook of cognitive-behavioral therapies* (pp. 357-386). New York: Guilford.

Mahoney, M., & Gabriel, T. J. (1987). Psychotherapy and cognitive sciences: An evolving alliance. *Journal of Cognitive Psychotherapy, 1*, 39-59.

Meichenbaum, D. (1985). *Stress-inoculation training*. New York: Pergamon Press.

Meichenbaum, D., & Gilmore, J. B. (1982). Resistance from a cognitive-behavioral perspective. In P. Wachtel (Ed.), *Resistance: Psychodynamic and behavioral approaches* (pp. 133-156). New York: Plenum.

Neimeyer, R. (1986). Personal construct therapy. In W. Dryden & W. Golden (Eds.), *Cognitive-behavioral approaches to psychotherapy* (pp. 224-260). New York: Harper and Row.

Padesky, C. (1988, Winter). Schema-focussed CT: Building new schemas. *International Cognitive Therapy Newsletter, 4*, 8-9.

Rehm, L. P. (1977). A self-control model of depression. *Behavior Therapy, 8*, 787-804.

Safran, J. D. (1984). Assessing the cognitive interpersonal cycle. *Cognitive Therapy and Research, 8*, 333-348.

Safran, J. D., & Segal, Z. V. (1990). *Cognitive therapy: An interpersonal perspective*. New York: Basic Books.

Weishaar, M., & Beck, A. T. (1986). Cognitive therapy. In W. Dryden & W. Golden (Eds.), *Cognitive-behavioral approaches to psychotherapy* (pp. 61-91). New York: Harper & Row.

# II

# Clinical Applications

# 4

# The Application of Cognitive Therapy to Patients with Personality Disorders

MARSHA M. ROTHSTEIN AND T. MICHAEL VALLIS

## INTRODUCTION

The demonstrated efficacy of cognitive therapy in the treatment of affective disorders (Hollon & Najavits, 1989; Murphy, Simons, Wetzel, & Lustman, 1984), anxiety disorders (Michelson & Ascher, 1987), eating disorders (Garner & Bemis, 1985; Wilson, 1986), and chronic pain (Turk, Meichenbaum, & Genest, 1983) has done much to legitimize cognitive therapy as a form of psychotherapy. As cognitive therapy has become more widely practiced, the types of patients referred to cognitive therapists have become more diverse. No longer is it true that cognitive therapists function largely in research or specialized treatment units. One of the more challenging issues faced by cognitive therapists is working with patients meeting the criteria for personality disorder (DSM-III-R; American Psychiatric Association, 1987).

In this chapter, adaptations of cognitive therapy required when working with this difficult patient population are outlined. Knowing how to adapt and implement cognitive therapy requires an understanding of who is being treated. Yet personality disorders represent a somewhat ambiguous population (witness the difficulty in achieving diagnos-

MARSHA M. ROTHSTEIN • Independent Practice, Delisle Court Professional Center, 1560 Yonge Street, Suite 300, Toronto, Ontario M4T 2S9, Canada.    T. MICHAEL VALLIS • Departments of Psychology and Psychiatry, Dalhousie University, and Department of Psychology, Camp Hill Medical Center, Halifax, Nova Scotia B3H 3G2, Canada.

tic reliability; Frances & Widiger, 1986; Garfield, 1986). In light of this ambiguity we briefly outline current conceptual and methodological issues regarding personality and personality disorders. Following this, existing cognitive therapy interventions with personality-disordered patients are critically reviewed. It is argued that, given the nature of personality disorders, the impact of existing cognitive therapy interventions is often limited. In such cases, a process-oriented approach to cognitive therapy may be more effective in facilitating therapeutic change. Development of dysfunctional self-beliefs, interpersonal schemata (Safran, 1988), and the meaning of the therapeutic relationship are central process variables in this approach.

## UNDERSTANDING PERSONALITY AND PERSONALITY DISORDERS

Millon (1986a) defines personality as "an inferred abstraction rather than a tangible phenomenon with material existence" (p. 642). He likens it to the body's physical systems and structures, composed of a tightly knit organization of traits and behaviors. Most personality theorists would agree that individuals possess relatively enduring personality traits during their lifetimes that distinguish them from others (Cloninger, 1987; Millon, 1986b).

The manifestation of personality traits is significantly influenced by the individual's environment. It is the interaction between psychological and biological characteristics within the social setting that determines the "character" of the individual (Bowlby, 1988; Cloninger, 1987). Such a biopsychosocial theory suggests that personality is not a static entity formed during childhood and stable over time, but a dynamic entity that unfolds over time. Understanding the reciprocal relationship between individuals and their environments is critical to an understanding of personality and personality disorders.

Personality theorists, in general, have adopted a dimensional model of personality. Two or three underlying dimensions, such as dominance and affiliation in interpersonal behavior, have usually been identified to describe personality (Horowitz & Vitkus, 1986). The work of Eysenck (1970) and Cloninger (1987) are good examples of this approach. Eysenck's work on neuroticism-psychoticism and introversion-extraversion is well known. Cloninger attempts to describe adaptive *and* maladaptive personality variants along the same dimensions and concludes that "the underlying structure of normal adaptive traits is the same as that of maladaptive traits" (p. 585). Widiger, Trull, Hunt, Clarkin, and

Frances (1987) reach similar conclusions, and they propose that the DSM-III-R personality disorders be differentiated on the basis of three higher-order dimensions: assertion (dominance), anxious rumination versus behavioral acting out, and social involvement (affiliation).

In contrast to the dimensional model of personality, diagnosis of personality disorder has been historically based on the classical model of categorization (Francis & Widiger, 1986). In this model, categories are considered as discrete entities, where the defining features are singly necessary and jointly sufficient, the boundaries between categories are distinct, and the members of each category are homogeneous (Cantor, Smith, French, & Mezzick, 1980). Examination of the DSM-III-R personality disorder criteria reflects this categorical approach. In DSM-III-R (APA, 1987), there are 11 separate personality disorder categories, with specific inclusion criteria for each. An individual either meets the criteria for a given disorder or does not. This presents a problem for patients who are dysfunctional but do not meet the inclusion criteria. The status of these patients vis-à-vis diagnosis and treatment is in question.

In recognition of the limits of the classical model of categorization of personality disorders, prototypes have been advocated as an alternative (Frances & Widiger, 1986; Millon, 1986a; Widiger et al., 1987). Prototypes describe a theoretical ideal or standard against which real people can be compared and consist of the most common features of members of a category (Millon, 1986a). Within a prototypal model, categories are not homogeneous, they do not have distinct boundaries, and defining characteristics vary in their validity (Frances & Widiger, 1986). Using this model, one can expect greater variability in presentation between individuals with the same personality disorder diagnosis, and greater overlap between diagnoses (i.e., a larger proportion of *mixed* personality disorders). One might also expect that the more prototypal an individual, the greater the reliability of that person's diagnosis. These conditions certainly appear to apply in clinical work with personality disorders. The increased variability that follows from a prototypal model of personality disorders implies that a highly idiographic approach is needed when working with this population.

Understanding personality disorders requires the differentiation of normal and pathological personality characteristics. Inflexibility, maladaptiveness, and functional/subjective distress are the criteria employed in the DSM-III and DSM-III-R to distinguish personality traits (normal) from personality disorders (pathological; DSM-III-R, 1987, p. 335). Millon (1986b) proposes three similar criteria to distinguish normal from pathological personality. These include: *functional inflexibility*, in which strategies for relating to others may be rigidly applied or applied when not appropriate; *self-perpetuation*, in which misconstrual of the world leads to further pathology; and *structural instability*, in which the individual reverts to old patterns and loses cognitive and emotional control under stress. Thus, not only do the different dimensions of personality disorders overlap, but there is considerable variability in the degree of pathology within a given dimension.

In summary, personality disorders represent a highly complex set of disorders. Personality disorders can best be conceptualized as prototypes, whose defining features are manifestations of the interaction between enduring biological and psychological traits and the environment. Further, the personality features that define individual personality disorders fall along a continuum of severity. The determination of normalcy or pathology can be guided by an assessment of characteristics such as functional inflexibility, self-perpetuation, distress, and structural instability (cohesion).

It is clear that severity varies within any given personality disorder category. It has also been suggested that the different personality disorder category prototypes differ in severity of disturbance (e.g., the prototypal histrionic personality disorder patient compared to the prototypal borderline personality disorder patient). Millon (1986b) suggests a severity dimension (across personality disorder categories) that can be used to guide treatment implementation. Millon gauged severity by the likelihood that in North American society "the personality style would be able to maintain its structural coherence and would be able to function in a rewarding manner" (p. 666).

The first and least severe category is characterized by a coherence of the sense of self and by the ability to relate to others in a relatively nonconflictual way. Millon includes the dependent, histrionic, narcissistic, and antisocial personality disorders in this category. Seen as more severe than the first, the second category is characterized by a lower level of structural cohesion. Within this category Millon characterizes the passive-aggressive, compulsive, schizoid, and avoidant personality disorders. According to his conceptualization of passive-aggressive and compulsive personality disorders, these individuals repeatedly undo or reverse their actions, a pattern which confirms their sense of inner division and lack of psychic consistency. The schizoid and avoidant personality disorders are judged at a midlevel of severity because of their disengagement from support systems, which denies them sources of nurturance and cognitive stability. Millon's final category, the most severe, includes the borderline, paranoid, and schizotypal disorders, where structural integration and psychic functioning are poor.

Millon's categorization of severity clusters is useful when one con-

siders implementing cognitive therapy. One would expect greater difficulty in successfully implementing cognitive therapy as one moves from
less to more severe categories. With greater difficulties in structural
cohesion, it is reasonable to expect problems in following through on the
tasks of cognitive therapy (e.g., self-monitoring, conducting experiments). In such cases, greater modification of the standard cognitive
therapy approach would likely be required to implement cognitive interventions. Although we are aware of no empirical data comparing the
efficacy of cognitive therapy with different personality disorder categories, clinical experience would suggest that the degree of structural cohesion would impact on the efficacy of cognitive therapy interventions.

## CURRENT COGNITIVE THERAPY APPROACHES
## TO TREATING PERSONALITY DISORDERS

Until recently, the application of cognitive therapy to personality
disorders has not been considered. Beck (1989) and Young (1987, 1989)
have presented preliminary models of the cognitive characteristics of
personality disorders to which existing cognitive therapy interventions
can be applied. In this context, the work of Turner (1989) and Linehan
(1989), who propose cognitive-behavioral models of borderline personality disorder (Linehan refers to her approach as dialectical behavior
therapy), is also noteworthy.

Beck and his colleagues (Beck, 1989; Weishaar, 1989) propose a
number of cognitive features to differentiate the personality disorders.
For each of the personality disorders they identify the following: view of
self, view of others, main belief, and main behavioral/interpersonal
strategy. To illustrate the differences between disorders, consider their
view of dependent and histrionic personality disorders. According to
Beck's scheme, individuals with dependent personality disorders view
themselves as needy, weak, helpless, and incompetent. They view others as nurturant, supportive, and competent, and have main beliefs
revolving around needing people to survive and to be happy, and needing a steady, uninterrupted flow of support and encouragement. Finally, their main coping strategy is to cultivate dependent relationships.
In contrast, individuals with histrionic personality disorders view themselves as glamorous and impressive, and view others as seducible, receptive, and admiring. Further, these individuals hold as main beliefs
the opinion that people are there to serve them and that others have no
right to deny them their wishes. Their major behavioral strategies include the use of charm and dramatic actions (such as temper tantrums,

suicide gestures) to achieve their goals. Using this model, Beck and his colleagues work to uncover the relevant cognitive characteristics and apply standard cognitive therapy interventions (e.g., dysfunctional thought records, behavioral experiments) to modify them (see Weishaar, 1989).

Young (1987, 1989) has also developed a cognitive model of personality disorders, called schema-focused cognitive therapy. Briefly, Young proposes that personality-disordered individuals can be characterized by the formation of early maladaptive schemata. Young proposes that such early maladaptive schemata can be differentiated from automatic thoughts, cognitive distortions, and underlying assumptions. Early maladaptive schemata are thought to be stable and enduring thought patterns that develop early in an individual's life and influence later functioning in a dysfunctional and self-perpetuating manner.

Young has identified eighteen early maladaptive schemata which revolve around five major areas of vulnerability: autonomy, connectedness, competence, reasonable expectations, and realistic limits. He then categorizes the DSM-III-R personality disorders according to areas of vulnerability (among the five) and early maladaptive schemata (among the eighteen). For example, the proposed area of vulnerability for compulsive personality disorder patients involves reasonable expectations, and the specific schemata include unrealistic standards, excessive self-control, and guilt/punishment. In contrast, with dependent personality disorders, the main proposed area of vulnerability involves autonomy, and specific associated schemata include vulnerability to harm/illness, dependence, subjugation/lack of individuation, and fear of losing emotional control.

The cognitive models of Beck and Young represent a significant advance in applying cognitive therapy to personality disorders. These models are particularly useful at a descriptive level, in the identification of cognitive features that potentially differentiate the various personality disorders. They are limited, however, in that there is no empirical evidence to date to validate their categorizations. If one accepts the notion of personality prototypes, then it is not clear how accurate the specific conceptualization of each personality disorder is. Specifically, it is not clear whether all patients, within a given personality disorder category, exhibit the same cognitive features. The degree of overlap between the cognitive features of each disorder is also unclear. A further limitation is that neither Beck's nor Young's model incorporates dimensions such as severity of disturbance, either within individual personality disorder categories, or between different categories. Not all individuals with personality disorders can be expected to respond to cognitive therapy, and it would be useful to identify criteria which might differentiate individuals who are either good or poor candidates for cognitive therapy.

The above issues notwithstanding, these models do identify relevant cognitive targets for intervention. Once relevant cognitive factors are identified, standard cognitive therapy interventions can be implemented to promote adaptive change. Unfortunately, standard cognitive therapy interventions are often limited in effectiveness. The successful implementation of standard cognitive interventions generally requires the following patient characteristics: ability to view their problem in a way that is (or becomes) compatible with the cognitive therapy rationale, a willingness to learn coping strategies, a willingness to accept the therapist as an educator, an ability to implement cognitive therapy techniques (e.g., collect evidence, role play, challenge negative thoughts), and an ability to follow a structured approach. However, the nature of personality disorders often precludes these conditions. Even when standard interventions work, their impact may be restricted by these factors as well.

In several recent studies, data have been reported which suggest that factors such as compatibility with the cognitive therapy rationale and willingness to accept the therapist as an educator influence the outcome of cognitive therapy within a depressed sample. Fennell and Teasdale (1987) examined a group of clinically depressed patients receiving a 20-session protocol of cognitive therapy (à la Beck, Rush, Shaw, & Emery, 1979). They divided the cognitive therapy group into rapid and slow responders. Rapid cognitive therapy responders displayed greater improvement (on the Beck Depression Inventory) by the second week of treatment and maintained this advantage throughout the treatment protocol, relative to slow responders. What is most interesting in this study is that Fennell and Teasdale were able to differentiate rapid and slow cognitive therapy responders on attitudinal variables. Rapid responders endorsed the cognitive therapy rationale to a significantly greater degree than slow responders, and rapid responders reported a more positive response to initial homework assignments. These data suggest that compatibility with the cognitive therapy rationale and attitude toward homework exercises may mediate the efficacy of cognitive therapy. A second study, by Persons, Burns, and Perloff (1988) reported on predictors of outcome and dropout in depressed patients treated with cognitive therapy (à la Beck et al., 1979) in a private practice setting. Persons et al. found that patients who completed homework assignments improved three times as much (using the Beck Depression Inventory) as those not completing the homework assignments. Further, they reported that the presence of a personality disorder was a significant predictor of premature termination of therapy. Collectively, these data confirm the importance of compatibility with the cognitive therapy rationale and willingness to perform the tasks of cognitive therapy (homework) as important process variables relating to outcome in depression. Yet, patients with personality disorders often have difficulty with these issues.

To illustrate the potential difficulties that can be encountered when implementing standard cognitive interventions with personality disorders, consider the following patient, who was seen by one of the authors for cognitive therapy.

> The patient, S.H., was a 36-year-old divorced mother who had been diagnosed as having a mixed dependent-avoidant personality disorder. S.H. had been experiencing a number of ongoing psychosocial stressors at the time of referral. These included increased demands at work, significant conflict with one daughter (tentatively diagnosed as a borderline personality disorder), and pervasive loneliness associated with a tendency to withdraw from all social contacts because of a fear of rejection. S.H. had experienced a major depression and was referred for cognitive therapy while she was an inpatient in a psychiatric unit.

The early phase of cognitive therapy followed closely the protocol of Beck *et al.* (1979). S.H. was asked to begin monitoring her activities and cognitions and was assigned mastery and pleasure exercises. However, she had extreme difficulty completing homework assignments. She was able to identify negative and anxiety-provoking automatic thoughts but was extremely reluctant to change her behavior. The therapist initially attempted to handle this by exploring cognitions associated with homework completion, but this proved nonproductive. S.H. would become increasingly distressed at such times. Any efforts by the therapist to focus on her cognitions were perceived by S.H. as attempts to reject her. She would then withdraw in the session and refuse to continue.

The therapist's direct probing and attempts to actively intervene at the level of cognitive content appeared to jeopardize the tenuous therapeutic relationship with S.H. The following exchange illustrates the process. S.H. was reporting on the contacts that she had with people following discharge from hospital. While she was involved in an ongoing battle with her oldest daughter, she did have a positive relationship with her son. She also had developed two positive relationships in the hospital and continued to socialize with these individuals in the week preceding this session.

> Pt: (visibly upset), "I can't cope, everyone criticizes me, all day, everyday."
>
> Tx: "When you think this way, how does it make you feel?"

PT: "Nothing I do is good enough, I'm tired of living my life this way."

Tx: "Let's look at how you're viewing this situation. Can you think of times over the past week when you've not been criticized by others?"

PT: "Everybody controls me, I feel like a nothing."

Tx: "It might help if you begin to examine your negative thoughts in more detail. You believe you are controlled and criticized by others, and this belief increases your distress and hopelessness, especially when you believe that it is 100 percent true, all of the time. Looking back over the week, were there any times when you were not controlled or criticized, or times when you felt accepted?"

PT: (Patient looks down, becomes withdrawn, says nothing).

Tx: "Can you tell me what you are thinking right now, you just withdrew from me."

PT: "Why do you want to reject me?"

Tx: "I'm not sure I understand what you mean."

PT: "You used to be warm and understanding, I thought you cared. But then you turn cold and businesslike."

Tx: "What am I doing that makes you think that?"

PT: "I don't know, you just seem cold. If you don't want to see me anymore, I understand, I'm used to being rejected."

Tx: "So, if I hear what you're saying, you're telling me that when I try to help you examine your negative thoughts you sense me backing away and that makes you think I am rejecting you."

PT: "I can't stand this anymore, I just want to leave" (at this point the therapist stops this intervention and discusses the meaning of the therapeutic relationship to the patient).

This interchange was typical for this patient. A consistent pattern developed in therapy which involved her disclosure of very distressing personal experiences, such as horrific past sexual abuse. Once she disclosed this information, she appeared to become hypervigilent to rejection. Any attempts to systematically examine her thoughts (e.g., through thought records, behavioral experiments, role play, all of which she refused to perform) were interpreted as confirming her belief that she was being rejected by the therapist. While this example represents an extreme reaction to a cognitive therapy intervention, it is a reaction which is not uncommon with personality-disordered patients. Given that hypersensitivity, isolation, and unwillingness to interact without certainty of being positively received are diagnostic criteria for avoidant personality disorder, such patients may be prone to problematic reactions to standard cognitive therapy interventions.

If one accepts the premise that personality-disordered patients, as a group, are likely to have difficulty with many of the tasks of cognitive therapy, and that this would negatively impact on treatment efficacy, two strategies could be adopted to resolve this problem. One strategy would be to select patients who are likely to benefit from cognitive therapy and refuse to treat those who do not meet these selection criteria. A second strategy would be to modify the cognitive therapy interventions to address the particular problems found with the personality disorders.

We are aware of no specific work with personality disorders that attempts to identify relevant selection criteria. However, Safran, Segal, Vallis, and Shaw (1990) have developed an interview-based suitability for cognitive therapy scale with anxious and depressed individuals that may be useful with personality-disordered individuals. Safran *et al.* use a semistructured interview to obtain ratings on 10 variables thought to relate to suitability for cognitive therapy. Items are rated on 5-point Likert-type scales (1 = negative prognosis, 5 = positive prognosis) and are as follows:

  1. Accessibility of automatic thoughts
  2. Awareness and differentiation of emotions
  3. Acceptance of personal responsibility for change
  4. Compatibility with cognitive therapy rationale
  5. Alliance potential—in session
  6. Alliance potential—out of session
  7. Chronicity of problems
  8. Security operations
  9. Focality
  10. Patient optimism/pessimism

Safran, Segal, Shaw, and Vallis (1990) have demonstrated that this scale can be rated reliably by experts (e.g., item intra-class correlation coefficients range from .46 to .98, with only one item having a reliability coefficient below .75). As well, the scale was predictive of outcome for short-term cognitive therapy for a mixed anxious-depressed group.

Provided that this scale demonstrates predictive validity within the personality disorder population, it could be used to select those personality-disordered patients likely to benefit from short-term cognitive therapy. However, given the nature of personality disorders, this approach may exclude the majority of individuals and leave only a minority who are highly appropriate for the standard cognitive therapy protocol. Few personality-disordered patients would be rated highly (suitable) on items such as chronicity, optimism, focality, security operations, or alliance potential.

As opposed to selecting those most suitable for the existing protocol, cognitive therapists might consider modifying their interventions to better suit the needs of the personality disordered. It is to this issue that we now turn.

## An Integrative Model of Cognitive Therapy for Personality Disorders

It has been argued that personality-disordered patients often have difficulty following through on many of the tasks of cognitive therapy. As such, cognitive therapy interventions may be best implemented in the context of a conceptual model that integrates technique with process variables (such as the development of dysfunctional self-beliefs, interpersonal schemata, and the meaning of the therapeutic relationship). This requires conceptual, procedural, and process adaptations of many common practices within cognitive therapy.

### Conceptual Adaptations Required

Most important in treating patients with personality disorders is the adoption of a model of cognitive therapy that is broad based. Cognitive therapy should be seen as an integrated, systemic form of psychotherapy, in which the central focus of therapy is on dysfunctional beliefs concerning the self and one's world, and in which the therapist's conceptualization focuses on cognitive processes, both conscious (automatic thoughts) and nonconscious (dysfunctional schemata; Turk & Salovey, 1985). As a system of psychotherapy, the cognitive therapist does not necessarily restrict his/her interventions to the cognitive or cognitive-behavioral domain. A wide range of interventions are used, and interventions may be selected (e.g., two-chair gestalt technique) on the basis of a consideration of a number of complex, situation-specific issues. What makes the approach cognitive is the conceptualization of the problem and the target of the intervention (i.e., a shift in dysfunctional cognitive processes).

In terms of conceptual models, we draw heavily on constructivist and interpersonal models of cognitive therapy, as illustrated by the work of Guidano and Liotti (1983), Mahoney (1989), and Safran and Segal (1990; see Chapter 1, this volume). Following the constructivist model, cognitive therapy involves the identification of underlying, deep (tacit) knowledge structures regarding the self and one's world (core schemata). Much work is devoted to a developmental analysis of the genesis of such cognitive structures. Interventions are more process based than technical, and are more focused on underlying cognitive structure (self-schemata) than on accessible automatic thoughts.

Integrating the constructivist model into cognitive therapy when treating personality-disordered patients has a number of advantages. First, there is increased *flexibility* that allows the therapist to more closely track the patient. Thus, interventions are timed according to patient receptivity. The standard cognitive therapy approach is structured to the point where interventions are often therapist generated. Second, there is greater attention placed on *developmental issues*. This has obvious relevance for personality-disordered patients whose problems are by definition longstanding and for whom early developmental experiences often play a major role in the genesis of their disorder (see Young, 1987). Third, greater attention is placed on the *process* of therapy, including the meaning of the therapeutic relationship itself. This allows a wide variety of problem issues such as trust, intimacy, and resistance to be addressed.

## Procedural Adaptations Required

Cognitive therapy is widely known to be a highly structured approach. Beck *et al.*'s (1979) cognitive therapy of depression and Meichenbaum's (1977) stress inoculation training are illustrations of this. The standard Beck cognitive therapy protocol is time limited, with the 20-session protocol being most common in evaluation studies.* Both the sequence and content of sessions tend to be structured. The typical course of cognitive therapy focuses initially on educational and behavioral interventions, then moves to an examination of thinking "errors" and distortions, and finally addresses dysfunctional assumptions. Individual sessions also tend to be structured around setting agendas, systematic examination of problem situations, feedback, and assigning homework.

While this structure can be an efficient and effective method for implementing cognitive therapy (as evidenced by available outcome studies; Rush, Beck, Kovacs, & Hollon, 1977; Blackburn, Bishop, Glen, Whalley, & Christie, 1981; Murphy *et al.*, 1984; Beck *et al.*, 1985), personality-disordered patients are likely to have difficulty with the structure of cognitive therapy (see above; Fennell & Teasdale, 1987;

---

*Persons, Burns, and Perloff (1988), in a study of predictors of dropout and outcome in cognitive therapy in a private practice sample, reported an average number of sessions of 18.39 for a sample of 70 patients. This is an important study because it is naturalistic. A standard limit on the number of sessions was not followed. Yet, on average, participants received the same number of sessions as with standardized protocols.

Persons *et al.*, 1988). Specifically, modification of the structure of cognitive therapy is required because patients with personality disorders often have great difficulty with issues such as compatibility with the cognitive therapy rationale, ability to implement homework exercises, and so on. The following structural adaptations are recommended. First, cognitive therapy should not be guided by a strict limit on the number of sessions. Although therapists must operate under the conditions of their settings (e.g., private practice versus hospital based), it is not reasonable to expect that significant change will occur in a predetermined number of sessions. Strict adherence to such a structure is likely to produce more problems than it solves. Patients might perceive themselves as inadequate because they are not responding as fast as they should, or therapists might perceive themselves as inadequate for the same reason. Second, the structure of an individual session should be guided by relevant process issues as opposed to any standard protocol. For example, it is common in cognitive therapy with a unipolar depressed patient to use the dysfunctional thought record to identify and reexamine several cognitive distortions within a session. With practice this process of identification and reevaluation becomes very efficient. In contrast, personality-disordered patients often are unable or unwilling to follow through on this process or to derive benefit from it. To persist at a task that the patient is unable to use will only detract from the working alliance.

## Process Adaptations Required

Finally, in adapting cognitive therapy to working with personality disorders special attention needs to be given to process issues. In general, the development and maintenance of a working therapeutic alliance with personality-disordered patients is tenuous. The therapist needs to be highly sensitive to the state of the alliance, and much work goes into establishing and maintaining a functional alliance (see Jacobson, 1989). For this reason the therapist should be prepared to deviate from ongoing interventions, in order to maintain the alliance. As a result, the timing of interventions is critical.

The relationship between the patient and therapist is a powerful therapeutic tool in all forms of cognitive therapy (Jacobson, 1989; Safran & Segal, 1990; Young, 1987; see Chapter 3, this volume) and is particularly so when working with personality disorders. The majority of patients suffering from personality disorders (e.g., avoidant, dependent, compulsive) have fundamental difficulties in how they relate to others. Also, it is common for such individuals to have not had a healthy relationship with another. As such, the therapy relationship can be the vehicle through which significant change in personal and interpersonal schemata (Safran & Segal, 1990) occurs.

In working with this population, resistance to change is a common and important therapeutic issue. As discussed in Chapter 3 (this volume), resistance can be more than a technical problem. An exploration of resistance as a form of self-protection can be productive with this patient group. Finally, it is important for the cognitive therapist to be aware of his/her own expectations in treating personality-disordered patients. Approaching such patients with the expectation that standard techniques will be effective can lead to significant frustration. As well, it is important to develop realistic goals based on the patient's personal resources, history of adaptive functioning, and biopsychosocial context.

## GUIDELINES FOR IMPLEMENTING AN INTEGRATIVE MODEL OF COGNITIVE THERAPY

In this section we will detail general strategies for implementing cognitive therapy with personality disorders and will illustrate these strategies with a case example. As discussed above, we advocate an integrative approach to therapy, in which technique and process interventions are combined to effect maximal change in dysfunctional cognitive content, process, and structure.

The implementation of cognitive therapy can be divided into two major phases. The first phase involves the development of a comprehensive cognitive *conceptualization* of the problem, and the second phase involves active *intervention strategies* that follow from this conceptualization. Each of these stages will be considered in turn. It should be noted that the conceptualization-intervention differentiation is somewhat arbitrary. Both processes occur simultaneously. Nonetheless, there is heuristic value in drawing a distinction between the activities. The case that will be presented is of a young man, D.S., who was diagnosed as having an avoidant personality disorder.

> D.S. is a 32-year-old single male postal worker who had sought help over the past three years for severe panic attacks, social withdrawal, and depression. Previous treatment included psychodynamic psychotherapy with a psychiatrist and a social worker, medication, and biofeedback/relaxation, all to no avail. At the time he was referred for cognitive therapy he led a very restricted life, in which he avoided almost all contact with people whenever possible. He avoided most social situations, including family gatherings, shopping malls, restaurants, and other public

places, and was extremely uncomfortable in work interactions (e.g., he avoided applying for job promotions because they required greater social contact). His life was restricted to going to work, travelling home, sleeping, and returning to work. D.S. clearly met the criteria for avoidant personality disorder, and in fact was highly prototypic of that disorder. Specifically, he demonstrated hypersensitivity to rejection, social withdrawal, unwillingness to enter relationships without guarantees of acceptance, low self-esteem, and desire for affection. These features had been highly characteristic of him over the past 10 years.

## Conceptualization Phase

In forming a conceptualization of a case it is essential to consider a number of issues (and their meaning). These issues include: *understanding the symptoms* presented by the patient, consideration of the *therapeutic process* and how it can be used in developing a comprehensive conceptualization, exploration of the *cognitive-developmental process*, and, finally, conceptualizing *core schemata*. Readers should consult Chapters 2 and 3 (this volume) for background information concerning the importance of conceptualization and the use of the therapeutic relationship in cognitive therapy. Given the long-standing functional difficulties associated with personality disorders, and the general resistance to treatment characteristic of this group, considerable time is often required in the conceptualization phase of treatment. Interventions need to be chosen carefully and timed such that the likelihood of change is maximized.

### Understanding Symptoms and Their Meaning

The symptoms experienced by the individual are usually the primary reason for his/her seeking help. Symptoms, therefore, are the initial focus in cognitive therapy. It is standard practice to conduct a meaning inquiry regarding reported symptoms. Therapists assess the accessible cognitions associated with the symptoms and examine these cognitions with respect to how functional/dysfunctional they are. By following normative models such as those of Beck (1989) or Young (1989), the therapist can identify key areas of vulnerability, and therefore, targets for change. Further, it is important to explore the meaning of these symptoms vis-à-vis the self and in this way obtain information regarding potential core cognitive processes (Guidano & Liotti, 1983; Safran, Vallis, Segal, & Shaw, 1986; Chapter 2, this volume). With respect to our case study:

> D.S.'s symptoms of anxiety were explored in detail by having him describe
> situations in which they occurred, using standard self-monitoring and

recording techniques. Automatic thoughts, such as "people will see I am nervous" and "this could lead to a full panic attack," were identified. The meaning of these thoughts was explored in detail on a number of occasions. The notion of being a "wimp" was a common response to such meaning inquiries and was associated with significant affect. Further exploration indicated that D.S. associated being a "wimp" with being weak and no good. This information helped the therapist conceptualize the construct "wimp" as central to D.S.'s view of himself. In any social situation at work or with friends, if he were to blush, he would automatically think "I am a wimp." This construct was connected to his belief that men had to be constantly in control of their emotions or otherwise they were weak and ineffectual. He considered himself as inadequate as a man because he was not in control of his emotions most of the time. Only as he began to identify those times that he was in control, or those times that other men were not, did he alter his view that an "adequate" man did not always have to be in control of his feelings.

In assessing meaning, it is also important to consider how an individual's symptoms fit into their affective and interpersonal domains. Symptoms and associated dysfunctional cognitions may have functional value for the patient. For instance, in a highly dependent individual self-effacing comments and helpless/hopeless beliefs may serve an interpersonal function, communicating to others that the individual is helpless. Direct intervention on these cognitions might be resisted due to an unwillingness to give up a dependent role. Greenberg and Safran (1987) refer to a similar process in their discussion of instrumental emotions. Instrumental emotions are seen to have some payoff or secondary gain, often interpersonal, associated with them. These instrumental emotions can be conceptualized as ineffective attempts at coping. Assessing the potential meaning of cognitions at an interpersonal level can be very useful in selecting therapeutic targets. Apparent dysfunctional cognitions that serve an interpersonal function (such as the histrionic who reports thoughts such as "I'm ugly" or "I'm not good enough" in situations where praise is likely) might best be dealt with by not directly challenging them. In this example, for instance, the therapist might not choose to encourage the patient to examine evidence for his/her beauty or competence but rather explore and challenge reasons why the patient requires praise from others. In summary, we recommend that with personality disorders, the cognitive therapist assess dysfunctional cognitions (automatic thoughts and cognitive distortions), obtain information relevant to core cognitive processes (as illustrated in the case of D.S.), and evaluate the potential interpersonal influences of these cognitive phenomena.

*Therapeutic Process*

It is all too easy for cognitive therapists to become so focused on cognitive interventions that they overlook the process issues in therapy. This is considered an oversight, particularly when working with personality-disordered patients. Personality-disordered patients most often have significant difficulty in their relationships to others, including the therapist. The therapeutic relationship provides an excellent context in which to examine and to intervene when dysfunctional interpersonal processes occur. Safran (1984; Safran & Segal, 1990) has written extensively on the interface between cognitive and interpersonal approaches. In examining the therapeutic process, the therapist should be attuned to the strength of the alliance and to issues related to the development or impairment of a good working alliance. Questions such as "How does the patient react to my suggestions/recommendations?" "How does he/she perceive our relationship?" and the like are important to keep in mind during the conceptualization phase of therapy. This information can often be used to help identify beliefs concerning the self and others, beliefs which often form the focus of the work with personality-disordered patients. In terms of our case example:

The initial stages of therapy were characterized by D.S.'s very cool, detached, rather cynical approach to therapy and the therapist. D.S. stated that this attempt at therapy was his last hope, but his behavior suggested that he did not really trust that it would work. This distrust, cynicism, lack of warmth, and discomfort in engaging with the therapist were selected as important therapeutic targets and were used to further explore D.S.'s beliefs about himself. However, the therapist decided that D.S. could not deal with an exploration of the therapeutic relationship until well after therapy had progressed, because D.S. needed to keep his distance as a means of self-protection. About eight months after therapy began, the opportunity did arise to use the therapeutic relationship as a means of understanding and dealing with D.S.'s avoidance of social contacts. After several agreements to call old friends, D.S. had still not done so. The therapist, upon questioning D.S.'s unwillingness to call his friends, learned that he believed it was pointless because he considered himself incapable of establishing a relationship of any kind—"I am unlikable." The therapist, by giving her impression about how the therapeutic relationship had progressed, helped D.S. explore the quality of the therapeutic relationship. D.S. admitted that he felt much more "connected" to the therapist than when he had begun therapy. He concluded that perhaps he was capable of establishing a relationship outside of therapy and the only way of finding out was to initiate contact with others, which he did.

*Cognitive-Developmental Process*

In developing a comprehensive conceptualization of a patient with a personality disorder, a third area that needs to be addressed is the relevant developmental issues which impact on the individual's current view of himself/herself. By definition, personality disorders are long-standing (DSM-III-R, 1987) and generally have their roots in early development (Bowlby, 1982, 1985). It is not at all uncommon for those with personality disorders to state that they have never had a positive view of themselves or their lives. As explicated by Guidano and Liotti (1983), exploration of a patient's developmental history provides the individual with an opportunity to, in an emotionally real manner, appreciate how his early experiences influenced his view of himself and his world. This process can be invaluable for producing a decentering, in which individuals are able to obtain a metaperspective on their cognitive processes. It is at such times when patients are often most amenable to change (Safran & Segal, 1990). With our case example:

> In an exploration of developmental issues, D.S. described his relationship with his parents as emotionally deprived. He felt that he could never count on his parents, who were devoutly religious, for emotional support. For example, he recounted that when he was 11 he returned home from school crying because his classmates had taunted him about the way he dressed. Rather than offering to help him, his parents suggested that he go to his room and pray. He realized then that his parents would not support him, and if he was to get along in the world it was solely up to him—he could trust no one. He was a very shy boy and found it excruciating to speak up in class or in a group of people. Ridiculed by his peers for his shyness, he developed the belief that the world was a threatening place and that his ability to cope within it was minimal. These three beliefs, which developed from experiences in childhood and adolescence (i.e., "The world is a threatening place," "I can't trust anyone to help me," and "I can't count on myself very well"), were critical for the therapist to know in conceptualizing his difficulties as an adult.

*Conceptualizing Core Schemata*

Once sufficient understanding of the patient and his/her difficulties occurs, such that the therapist understands the symptoms, the nature of the treatment process, and relevant developmental issues, this information should be constructed into a formal conceptualization. Conceptualization should be hierarchical in nature, such that hypotheses are generated as to peripheral and core cognitive processes.

The assessment and conceptualization of core schemata is a highly idiosyncratic process, which takes into account the particular circumstances of the individual, how these circumstances are perceived by him/her, and how they affect him/her. We emphasize this process because it is important that the conceptual model that guides the therapist be explicitly stated (see Chapter 2, this volume). As indicated by Turk and Salovey (1985, among others), there are a variety of systematic biases that guide the judgments and inferences made by the clinician. Biases such as the confirmatory bias (the tendency to pay more attention to information consistent with one's bias), the availability heuristic (the tendency to make frequency judgments on the basis of ease of recall of events), or illusory correlation (the tendency to attribute causality between two events which coexist but in fact are unrelated) are unavoidable. In order to minimize the effects of such biases clinicians need to become aware of their inferences, how these inferences can be biased, and take steps to correct the bias. Turk and Salovey (1985) outline some strategies for debiasing the clinician. We argue that one of the best methods for facilitating this is to clearly state one's conceptualization and look for evidence to justify or refute it. In addition, "checking out" one's hypothesis with the patient by saying, for example, "Does this seem true for you or am I mistaken here?" would be another way of evaluating the therapeutic utility of one's conceptualization.

It should be obvious that the process of conceptualization, which is an assessment process, is a detailed and time-consuming one. For this reason, brief time-limited therapy can often be ineffective with personality-disordered patients. This is not to imply that one does not intervene until a clear conceptualization is formed. Quite the opposite. It is often through failed interventions that one identifies and diagnoses a personality disorder. It should be emphasized, however, that personality-disordered patients are complex, and therefore therapists should be prepared to examine in depth the nature of patients' cognitive organization and how this organization relates to personality style.

We are recommending, then, that when patients with personality disorders are treated in cognitive therapy, the therapist focuses his/her initial work on the development of a clear conceptualization. Standard techniques such as self-monitoring and attempting behavioral changes are important, but are not the sole defining characteristics of this early work. Instead, the bulk of the initial therapeutic effort is committed to helping the individual identify, appreciate, and reevaluate core dysfunctional processes. To return to our case, the following conceptualization was formulated:

> As a child, D.S's emotional needs were not met by his parents. If he was compliant, some positive comments were made but rarely was affection

demonstrated. He also learned in school that compliance meant not having negative attention drawn to him. Awareness of his parents' lack of social ease and teasing at school led to his beliefs that others were basically unkind and untrustworthy. Self-reliance became his only way of coping but proved to be ineffective because he saw himself as compliant, nonassertive, and emotionally weak. The panic attacks and avoidance of most social situations are understandable in light of these core constructs.

Given this conceptualization, therapy focused on changing core schemata about D.S. and his world. It was anticipated that helping him integrate new knowledge about himself as a capable person and about the world as relatively nonthreatening would go a long way in altering his beliefs about himself and the world. The therapeutic process was expected to be characterized by his lack of trust, and the therapist intended to use the therapeutic relationship as a tool to help D.S. change his beliefs about the danger of trusting others. In this way intervention targets were selected in a highly idiosyncratic manner that relied on a detailed conceptualization.

## Intervention Phase

We have noted previously that the conceptualization and the intervention phases in cognitive therapy are not necessarily distinct phases. Implementation of intervention strategies can be a means to test hypotheses that arise from an initial conceptualization of the patient's problems. The results of these interventions can enhance conceptualization, which in turn can lead to more effective interventions. Notwithstanding this interrelationship, we will discuss intervention strategies separately for clarification purposes.

The process of implementing intervention strategies consists of an *exploration* of the patient's thoughts, beliefs, and assumptions, the patient's core and peripheral cognitions, the affect-cognition relationship, and the capacity of the patient to decenter. *Interventions per se* include standard cognitive-behavior change strategies, as well as the use of the therapeutic relationship, and the patient's developmental context.

### Exploration

An examination of the patient's automatic thoughts, assumptions, and beliefs is one of the first steps in formulating effective interventions. Consider our case study:

When D.S. found himself in a social situation his *automatic thoughts* were: "It's terrible if I blush because people will know that I'm nervous" and "Oh no! I'm getting hot—I must be having an anxiety attack." Some of his *assumptions* were: "Most people don't like quiet people so they won't like me" and "Women expect boyfriends to be extroverted and sociable which I am not, so I'll never make it with a woman." Examples of his *beliefs* were: "I am a contemptible person because I am so weak" and "I am unlovable."

Following an examination of the patient's automatic thoughts, assumptions, and beliefs, a differentiation of those that are core and those that are peripheral can aid in selecting relevant targets of intervention. As noted above, this involves a vertical exploration of meaning vis-à-vis the self (Safran *et al.*, 1986). Consider the following exchange with D.S. as an illustration of this:

PT: "I'm afraid to meet new people because I may blush."

TX: "What other thoughts do you have when you meet strangers?" (horizontal exploration)

PT: "They'll see that I'm nervous and most people don't like nervous people."

TX: "What does it mean for you to blush?" (vertical exploration)

PT: "It means that I'm weak, a nerd, not emotionally strong."

TX: "When you say this about yourself how do you feel about yourself?"

PT: "I feel terrible. I feel like a wimp—a nothing."

TX: "So when you blush you end up thinking that you are weak, worthless?"

PT: "Yes." (visibly upset, head bowed)

An assessment of the relationship between affect and cognition in cognitive therapy is important because it is often through feelings that patients come to an understanding of self (Guidano & Liotti, 1983; Greenberg & Safran, 1987). Core cognitions can often result from an exploration of the patient's emotions in therapy. In our case study:

When D.S. expressed his dissatisfaction with his social life he appeared quite sad. When asked how he was feeling, D.S. admitted to his sadness and said "I have to endure too much—I guess I just have a depressed personality." By exploring his feelings of sadness the therapist was able to access a central self-concept that impeded his sense of competency and control. Intervention strategies could then be formulated to deal with this issue.

The final area to explore when devising intervention strategies is the patient's capacity to decenter. If patients cannot distance themselves somewhat from their difficulties and their perception of these difficulties (i.e., obtain a metaperspective), interventions may be needed to help them gain a more objective perspective. For example, in our case study:

> The therapist's initial attempts to help D.S. take a less personal view of his problems led to many "yes . . . but . . . " responses. However, in one of the early therapy sessions the following interchange took place:
>
> Pt: "Other men are usually very confident, and extroverted."
>
> Tx: "Have you ever seen other men like yourself who are quiet at parties?"
>
> Pt: "Yes, but they don't look nervous like I do."
>
> Tx: "You mean, you've never seen other men at parties who look nervous?"
>
> Pt: "Well yes, but I know they aren't as nervous as I am—besides I don't really care about them—it's me. I don't want to be nervous."
>
> Tx: "You mean, even though other men do appear nervous at parties and that's ok—you could never allow yourself to look nervous."
>
> Pt: "Yeah—I guess I'm looking for perfection for myself—maybe I really can't be all that I think I should be."
>
> This comment informed the therapist that the patient was able to decenter somewhat.

### Intervention

We recommend the following intervention strategies in the treatment of personality disorders: the examination of *developmental issues* to facilitate reappraisal of self-schemata, the use of the *therapeutic relationship* to facilitate reappraisal of self- and interpersonal schemata, and *standard cognitive behavior change strategies.*

By examining *developmental processes*, the patient can begin to understand the history of his/her core cognitions. This understanding then allows the patient to reappraise his/her self-knowledge in light of the here and now. For example, in our case study:

> Through an exploration of his negative experiences in public school and his poor relationship with his parents, D.S. came to understand his sense of himself as weak and unassertive. By having him describe his present abilities to take care of himself physically and emotionally, he was able to reappraise himself as no longer the helpless, weak little boy that he was but as a mature, competent man. This intervention extended over a number of sessions, and the therapist encouraged D.S. to repeatedly enumerate and act upon his current self-care skills. As his ability to influence events became more apparent to him, he became more willing to reappraise and challenge his view of himself as weak.

In Chapter 3 (this volume), the *therapeutic relationship* was described as a useful intervention tool. This is particularly true for personality disorders, where interpersonal issues such as trust, intimacy, and control are often central to these patients' difficulties. Therapy can be the one safe place for the patient to examine interpersonal schemata (see Mahoney, 1989). With respect to our case study:

> It took several months for D.S. even to engage in small talk with the therapist at the beginning and end of each session. Eventually, the therapist was able to use humor to help him decenter. It took almost a year before the therapist could use the relationship as a means of challenging some of D.S.'s beliefs about himself. When the therapist questioned him about the importance of the therapeutic relationship, D.S. countered, "Just the word—relationship—makes me uncomfortable." Over time, D.S. came to understand that if he could trust and be open emotionally with the therapist, perhaps he was capable of having a close relationship outside of therapy. The use of the therapeutic relationship to reappraise core constructs such as "I am unlikable" was a critical intervention with D.S.

Finally, *standard cognitive and behavior change strategies* are an important part of the intervention process.* These include thought monitoring, behavioral experiments, use of dysfunctional thought records, role play, and so on (see Beck, 1989; Beck *et al.*, 1979; Weishaar, 1989; Young, 1989). Behavior change strategies help to alleviate symptoms like anxiety or depression and can lead to new self-knowledge, which when integrated into the self-schemata can lead to lasting change. In our case example:

> Behavioral and cognitive strategies were employed to help D.S. deal with his anxiety. A reduction of anxiety in social situations occurred when relaxation and cognitive reappraisal strategies were applied. For example, D.S. wished to attend a seminar but was terrified that he would have an anxiety attack in the auditorium. He spent some time in therapy practicing relaxation techniques and reappraising the situation if he did have anxiety (i.e., would people really notice and think he was a wimp, and what if they did). The first time he went to the seminar he became so anxious

---

*In this chapter we do not focus on standard cognitive and behavior change strategies for several reasons. This chapter is intended for cognitive therapists already familiar with standard cognitive therapy interventions but unfamiliar with how to adapt these techniques to working with patients with personality disorders. Further, there are a plethora of texts available to interested readers on implementing standard cognitive techniques (e.g., Beck, 1989; Beck *et al.*, 1979; Young, 1987). Finally, our intent has been to highlight process adaptations as opposed to content adaptations.

going through the auditorium door that he turned around and left. He returned the following week, and sat through the lectures, saying to himself, "Even if I do feel uncomfortable, this will pass" and "I'll just sit through it, the agony won't last forever." He managed to sit through the lecture with relative ease by relaxation techniques and self-talk. He felt enormously satisfied with his accomplishment. This type of change led to D.S. reappraising his belief that he was not in control of his life. New constructs of self-efficacy were introduced, which facilitated his growing sense of self-worth.

## SUMMARY

In this chapter, we have attempted to outline an integrative, process-based approach to cognitive therapy for personality-disordered patients. We endorse a prototypal approach to personality disorders, in which individuals vary in the extent to which they clearly meet the criteria for a given diagnosis. Such an approach to classification mandates approaching cognitive therapy in a highly idiographic manner.

Although there is little systematic work available on cognitive therapy for personality disorders, Beck and Young have each proposed content-based descriptions of the cognitive features of the different disorders. The model we propose is complementary to these content-based models and emphasizes conceptual, procedural, and process modifications required when conducting cognitive therapy with this group. We argue that such modifications are necessary since personality-disordered patients commonly have difficulty benefiting from cognitive interventions applied in a standard fashion. Finally, we have attempted to illustrate the procedures in conceptualizing and intervening by presenting, in detail, a case history of an individual with avoidant personality disorder. In particular, we emphasize the importance of a cognitive therapy approach that combines standard techniques with process-based interventions, particularly with the exploration of cognitive-developmental issues, interpersonal schemata, and the meaning of the therapeutic relationship.

## REFERENCES

American Psychiatric Association. (1987). Diagnostic and statistical manual of mental disorders (3rd ed., rev.). Washington, DC: Author.
Beck, A. T. (1989). Cognitive therapy of personality disorders: Introduction. Paper presented at the World Congress of Cognitive Therapy, Oxford, England.

Beck, A. T., Rush, A. J., Shaw, B. F., & Emery, G. (1979). *Cognitive therapy of depression*. New York: Guilford.

Beck, A. T., Hollon, S. D., Young, J. P., Bedrosian, R. C., & Budenz, D. (1985). Treatment of depression with cognitive therapy and amitriptyline. *Archives of General Psychiatry, 42*, 142-148.

Blackburn, I. M., Bishop, S., Glen, A. I. M., Whalley, L. T., & Christie, J. E. (1981). The efficacy of cognitive therapy in depression: A treatment trial using cognitive therapy and pharmacotherapy, each alone, and in combination. *British Journal of Psychiatry, 139*, 181-189.

Bowlby, J. (1982). *Attachment and loss, Vol. 1*. New York: Basic Books.

Bowlby, J. (1985). The role of childhood experience in cognitive disturbance. In M. Mahoney & A. Freeman (Eds.), *Cognition and Psychotherapy* (pp. 181-200). New York: Plenum.

Bowlby, J. (1988). Developmental psychiatry comes of age. *American Journal of Psychiatry, 145*:(1), 1-10.

Cantor, N., Smith, E., French, R. D., & Mezzick, J. (1980). Psychiatric diagnosis as a prototype categorization. *Journal of Abnormal Psychology, 89*, 81-89.

Cloninger, R. (1987). A systematic method for clinical description and classification of personality variants. *Archives of General Psychiatry, 44*, 573-588.

Eysenck, H. (1970). A dimensional system of psychodiagnostics. In A. Maher (Ed.), *New approaches to personality classifications* (pp. 169-207). New York: Columbia University Press.

Fennell, M., & Teasdale, J. (1987). Cognitive therapy for depression: Individual differences and the process of change. *Cognitive Therapy and Research, 11*, 253-272.

Frances, A., & Widiger, T. (1986). Methodological issues in personality disorder diagnosis. In T. Millon & G. Klerman (Eds.), *Contemporary directions in psychopathology: Towards the DSM-IV* (pp. 381-400). New York: Guilford.

Garfield, S. L. (1986). Problems in diagnostic classification. In T. Millon & G. Klerman (Eds.), *Contemporary directions in psychopathology: Toward the DSM-IV* (pp. 99-114). New York: Guilford.

Garner, D. M., & Bemis, K. M. (1985). Cognitive therapy for anorexia nervosa. In D. M. Garner & P. E. Garfinkel (Eds.), *Handbook of psychotherapy for anorexia and bulimia* (pp. 107-146). New York: Guilford.

Greenberg, L. S., & Safran, J. D. (1987). *Emotions in psychotherapy*. New York: Guilford.

Guidano, V. F., & Liotti, G. (1983). *Cognitive processes and emotional disorders: A structural approach to psychotherapy*. New York: Guilford.

Hollon, S. D., & Najavits, L. (1989). Review of empirical studies on cognitive therapy. In A. Frances & R. Hales (Eds.), *Review of psychiatry: Volume 7* (pp. 643-666). New York: American Psychiatric Press.

Horowitz, L. M., & Vitkus, J. (1986). The interpersonal basis of psychiatric symptoms. *Clinical Psychology Review, 6*, 443-470.

Jacobson, N. S. (1989). The therapist-client relationship in cognitive behavior therapy: Implications for treating depression. *Journal of Cognitive Psychotherapy: An International Quaterly, 3*, 85-96.

Linehan, M. M. (1989). Cognitive and behavior therapy for borderline personality disorder. *Annual review of psychiatry, Vol. 8* (pp. 84-102). Washington, DC: American Psychiatric Association.

Mahoney, M. J. (1989). The cognitive sciences and psychotherapy: Patterns in a developing relationship. In K. S. Dobson (Ed.), *Handbook of cognitive behavioral therapies* (pp. 357-386). New York: Guilford.

Meichenbaum, D. (1977). *Cognitive-behavior modification*. New York: Plenum.

Michelson, L., & Ascher, L. M. (1987). *Anxiety and stress disorders: Cognitive-behavioral assessment and treatment*. New York: Guilford.

Millon, T. (1986a). Personality prototypes and their diagnostic criteria. In T. Millon & G. Klerman (Eds.), *Contemporary directions in psychopathology: Towards the DSM-IV* (pp. 671-712) New York: Guilford.

Millon, T. (1986b). A theoretical derivation of pathological personalities. In T. Millon & G. Klerman (Eds.), *Contemporary directions in psychopathology: Towards the DSM-IV* (pp. 639-669). New York: Guilford.

Murphy, G. E., Simons, A. D., Wetzel, R. D., & Lustman, P. J. (1984). Cognitive therapy and pharmacotherapy, singly and together in the treatment of depression. *Archives of General Psychiatry, 41*, 33-41.

Persons, J. B., Burns, D. D., & Perloff, J. M. (1988). Predictors of dropout and outcome in cognitive therapy for depression in a private practice setting. *Cognitive Therapy and Research, 12*, 557-576.

Rush, A. J., Beck, A. T., Kovacs, M., & Hollon, S. D. (1977). Comparative efficacy of cognitive therapy and pharmacotherapy in the treatment of depressed out-patients. *Cognitive Therapy and Research, 1*, 17-37.

Safran, J. D. (1984). Assessing the cognitive-interpersonal cycle. *Cognitive Therapy and Research, 8*, 333-348.

Safran, J. D. (1988). *A refinement of cognitive behavioral theory and practice in light of interpersonal theory*. Clarke Institute of Psychiatry, Toronto.

Safran, J. D., & Segal, Z. V. (1990). *Cognitive therapy: An interpersonal process perspective*. New York: Basic Books.

Safran, J. D., Vallis, T. M., Segal, Z. V., & Shaw, B. F. (1986). Assessment of core cognitive processes in cognitive therapy. *Cognitive Therapy and Research, 10*, 509-526.

Safran, J. D., Segal, Z. V., Shaw, B. F., & Vallis, T. M. (1990). Patient selection for short-term cognitive therapy. In J. D. Safran & Z. V. Segal, *Interpersonal processes in cognitive therapy*. New York: Basic Books.

Safran, J. D., Segal, Z. V., Vallis, T. M., & Shaw, B. T. (1990). Suitability for short-term cognitive interpersonal therapy: Interview and rating scales. In J. D. Safran & Z. V. Segal, *Interpersonal processes in cognitive therapy*. New York: Basic Books.

Turk, D., & Salovey, P. (1985). Cognitive structures, cognitive processes, and cognitive-behavior modification: II. Judgements and inferences of the clinician. *Cognitive Therapy and Research, 9*, 19-34.

Turk, D., Meichenbaum, D., & Genest, M. (1983). *Pain and behavioral medicine: A cognitive-behavioral perspective*. New York: Guilford.

Turner, S. M. (1989). Case study evaluations of a bio-cognitive-behavioral approach for the treatment of borderline personality disorder. *Behavior Therapy, 20*, 477-489.

Weishaar, M. E. (1989). *Cognitive therapy of histrionic and passive-aggressive personality disorders*. Paper presented at the World Congress of Cognitive Therapy, Oxford, England.

Widiger, T., Trull, T., Hurt, S., Clarkin, J., & Frances, A. (1987). A multidimensional scaling of the DSM-III personality disorders. *Archives of General Psychiatry, 44*, 557-563.

Wilson, G. T. (1986). Cognitive-behavioral and pharmacological therapies for bulimia. In K. D. Brownell & J. P. Foreyt (Eds.), *Handbook of eating disorders: Physiology, psychology, and treatment of obesity, anorexia, and bulimia* (pp. 450-475). New York: Basic Books.

Young, J. E. (1987). *Schema-focused cognitive therapy for personality disorders*. Unpublished manuscript, Columbia University.

Young, J. E. (1989). *The role of interpersonal strategies in schema-focused cognitive therapy for personality disorders*. Paper presented at the World Congress of Cognitive Therapy, Oxford, England.

# 5

# *The Application of Cognitive Therapy to Posttraumatic Stress Disorder*

CAROL A. PARROTT AND JANICE L. HOWES

## OVERVIEW

In the present chapter, cognitive therapy for posttraumatic stress disorder (P.T.S.D.) in response to life-threatening trauma is outlined. The history of traumatic stress disorders is briefly discussed, followed by the current definition of P.T.S.D. (DSM-III-R; American Psychiatric Association, 1987). Etiological factors, and the role of pretrauma and posttrauma factors, are considered in the conceptualization of posttraumatic stress disorder. The focus of the chapter is on the phenomonological experience of trauma for the P.T.S.D. victim. The following cognitive issues are highlighted: appraisal of trauma, generalized belief of vulnerability, self-questioning, and self-appraisal. The implementation of cognitive therapy with P.T.S.D. victims is then explicated. Specific issues discussed include flexibility, resistance, therapeutic relationship, and acknowledgment and support. Case examples are used to illustrate a flexible cognitive therapy approach to the treatment of this disorder. Most of the clinical examples discussed are taken from the injured worker population.

CAROL A. PARROTT • Private Practice, 1060 Springhill Drive, Mississauga, Ontario L5H 1M9, Canada.    JANICE L. HOWES • Department of Psychiatry, Dalhousie University, and Department of Psychology, Camp Hill Medical Center, Halifax, Nova Scotia B3H 3G2, Canada.

## HISTORY AND INCIDENCE

Clinicians have identified, described, and treated stress disorders following trauma for many years. At the end of the nineteenth century and in the early twentieth, the development of Worker's Compensation Acts resulted in increased interest in posttraumatic disorders. Similarly, the American Civil War and World Wars I and II led to increased focus on posttraumatic sequelae. Terms like "nervous shock" and "compensation neurosis" appeared in the late nineteenth century to describe the emotional sequelae and invalidism of survivors of railway accidents (Trimble, 1985). "Shell shock," "war neurosis," "battle fatigue," and "war stress" were used to describe the psychological problems experienced by traumatized World War I and World War II veterans. "Survivor syndrome" has been used to refer to the long-standing psychological sequelae of survivors of concentration camps and hostage takings. Disorders in response to specific traumas have also been identified (e.g., rape trauma syndrome; Trimble, 1985). In the 1970s, the psychological problems displayed by Vietnam veterans were recognized and referred to as "Vietnam Stress Syndrome" and "Post-Vietnam Syndrome" (Thienes-Hontos, Watson, & Kucala, 1982). The term "posttraumatic neurosis" was also commonly used and was a harbinger of things to come in that a common syndrome, following varying traumatic situations and events, was recognized.

The term *posttraumatic stress disorder* was introduced in the third edition of the Diagnostic and Statistical Manual of Mental Disorders (DSM-III; American Psychiatric Association, 1980). The development of this diagnostic category has allowed the conceptualization of a syndrome which can encompass the multiple disorders previously referred to in the literature. This has heuristic value by facilitating standardization in the study of P.T.S.D. This term also has clear psycho-legal implications.

In DSM-III-R (American Psychiatric Association, 1987), posttraumatic stress disorder is regarded as an anxiety disorder. The necessary criteria for diagnosis include the following four characteristics. First, there must be a traumatic event, which is "outside the range of the usual human experience" and "would be markedly distressing to almost anyone" (p. 250). The clinical limitations of this concept with respect to the subjective experience of a traumatic event will be addressed later in the chapter. Second, there is persistent reexperiencing of the trauma through recurrent nightmares, intrusive recollections, reliving the trauma, flashbacks, hallucinations, and intense distress upon exposure to events symbolizing or resembling some aspect of the trauma. Third, there is numbing of general responsiveness to the external world (i.e., psychic numbing) or avoidance of stimuli related to the trauma. Fourth, a variety of autonomic, dysphoric, and cognitive symptoms suggestive of increased arousal are present. Phobic anxiety toward the traumatic stimuli is common. Recent research by Solomon (1988) suggests that P.T.S.D. is also associated with higher rates of somatic complaints.

The onset of the disorder is usually immediate but may be delayed (i.e., six months after the trauma). Delayed onset is more likely to be misdiagnosed if the traumatic event is not represented in the recent personal experience of the victim. In cases of delayed onset of P.T.S.D., the intensity of symptoms can increase with continued exposure to the traumatic stimulus. For example, a 30-year-old truck driver, who was involved in a motor vehicle accident in which a child was fatally injured, continued to function and drive his truck for several months but with increasing anxiety symptoms, fearfulness of driving, and more frequent and dysfunctional nightmares, flashbacks, and ruminations about the fatal accident. After 6 months, a full blown P.T.S.D. developed.

The degree of impairment displayed by individuals with P.T.S.D. ranges from mild to severe and may be complicated by interpersonal difficulties. Although some stress disorders resolve relatively quickly, a great many do not, and symptoms continue for years (e.g., Vietnam veterans can display symptoms many years following combat exposure; Stretch, 1986). Alternatively, aggravation of acute symptoms may occur after latency periods of months or years. The chronicity of posttraumatic stress symptoms is supported by Eitinger's (1969, cited in Marks, 1987) and Nadler and Ben-Shushan's (1989) findings with concentration camp survivors.

Most of the research on P.T.S.D. has focused primarily on soldiers with combat exposure, and especially on the experience of Vietnam veterans. The incidence of war-related P.T.S.D. in this latter group is high, and estimates range from 18% to 54% of veterans now in the civilian community (Stretch, Vail, & Maloney, 1985). Further statistics reveal that only 10.9% of U.S. Army Reserve Vietnam veterans and 5.1% of active duty Vietnam veterans display P.T.S.D. These differences in incidence rates are most likely related to support and selection factors. Stretch (1990) has recently completed a study comparing Canadian and U.S. Vietnam veterans, in which he found the rate of chronic P.T.S.D. to be 2.3 times higher for Canadian veterans than U.S. veterans. He considered the difference to be largely due to less social support and recognition in Canada, as well as less support from the government in terms of medical and psychological services.

There are limited incidence data for non-Vietnam veteran groups, particularly for individual victimization experiences. Although statistics for P.T.S.D. *per se* are rare, there is evidence that traumatic victimization experiences (e.g., rape, robbery, assault) do lead to serious risk for emotional disturbance (Kilpatrick *et al.*, 1985), as does exposure to natural disasters (e.g., Madakasira & O'Brien, 1987). Helzer, Robins, and McEvoy's (1987) study examining the incidence of P.T.S.D. in individuals in a major American city suggests that approximately 1% of the general population may display P.T.S.D. Further, Keane (1989) suggests that the incidence in the adult population may be as high as 2%. One of the difficulties in collecting incidence data for nonveteran groups, such as motor vehicle accident and industrial accident victims, is the frequent failure to recognize and diagnose traumatic stress symptoms.

## Etiology and Conceptualization

The most influential conceptual models of P.T.S.D. have been the behavioral model and the information-processing model, although biological models have also been proposed. *Behavioral models* of the development of P.T.S.D. derive from basic conditioning theory (Keane, Fairbank, Caddell, Zimering, & Bender, 1985a). The life-threatening trauma is viewed as the unconditioned stimulus, and the physiological arousal as the unconditioned response. Through higher-order conditioning, coexisting environmental and internal stimuli elicit physiological responses, and generalization occurs. Barlow (1988) describes the etiological process as "learned alarm." Intense emotions of fear, anxiety, and rage are "true alarms" experienced during exposure to a traumatic life event. A fear or anxiety response may then occur with stimuli which symbolize or are similar to some aspect of the event. This is a learned alarm. Learned helplessness may also play a central role in the development of P.T.S.D. (Seligman, 1975; Wilson, Smith, & Johnson, 1985).

Horowitz (1986) introduced the *information-processing* model of the stress response. According to Horowitz, a traumatic life event is processed and integrated into existent self-schemata through a "completion tendency." Outcry, avoidance, repetitive recollections, and reexperiencing are part of this process. Symptomatic numbing is seen as a defense. Patients may experience cyclical fluctuations between stages of avoidance and ruminations during the process of integrating the traumatic event into existent self-schemata. Litz and Keane (1989) have recently explicated information-processing factors that may contribute to the formation and maintenance of P.T.S.D. symptoms. Storage, retrieval, accessibility of the trauma (fear-related information), and attentional factors are all seen as playing a role in this process. It is suggested that fear-related information about the trauma is stored in a multidimensional fear network. Although memories may be avoided, either consciously or unconsciously, retrieval cues such as mood state or related environmental stimuli may activate fear-related information. Consistent with this, individuals with P.T.S.D. appear to attend to trauma-related cues in a biased manner (Litz & Keane, 1989). Finally, *biological* or biochemical etiological models are being proposed. It has been suggested that persistent changes may occur in the adrenergic system (during exposure) from prolonged hyperstimulation (Keane, 1988), or that the trauma results in dysregulation of noradrenergic systems (Krystal *et al.*, 1989). However, pharmacological treatment studies are few and generally have not supported the effectiveness of specific medications (Birkhimer, DeVance, & Muniz, 1985). The general pharmacological approach appears to be to medicate for the primary symptoms (e.g., antidepressants for depression).

A broader conceptual framework for P.T.S.D. involves an examination of *pre- and posttrauma factors*, as well as characteristics of the traumatic event itself. Research has been inconclusive with respect to predisposing factors such as personality or psychiatric history. For example, McFarlane (1988) collected data on a group of fire fighters exposed to a bushfire disaster and found a significant association between past personal or family history of psychiatric disorder and the development of chronic P.T.S.D. On the other hand, Hyer *et al.* (1986) found that premorbid adjustment problems or personality problems were not characteristic of war veterans who developed P.T.S.D. Foy, Sipprelle, Rueger, and Carroll (1984) reported no differences in premilitary adjustment between veterans with and without P.T.S.D. In a sample of injured workers with P.T.S.D. (Howes & Parrott, in review), we found that only 19% of our sample reported a history of psychological or psychiatric problems. Collectively, these data suggest that premorbid psychological problems are not necessary for the development of P.T.S.D. However, preexisting life events or pathology (e.g., previous anxiety or depressive disorder) may increase vulnerability in some cases.

Two major factors which seem related to the development and maintenance of P.T.S.D. in veterans are combat exposure (e.g., Barrett & Mizes, 1988; Foy *et al.*, 1984) and social support posttrauma. Several studies have highlighted the beneficial role of high levels of social support during the first year post-Vietnam (Barrett & Mizes, 1988; Foy *et al.*, 1984; Keane, Scott, Chavoya, Lamparski, & Fairbank, 1985b; Stretch, 1985). Similarly, Nadler and Ben-Shushan (1989) found that Holocaust survivors living in a kibbutz were better adjusted than those living in cities. Instrumental support and psychological support were the most frequently mentioned reasons for improved coping in the kibbutz. Other aspects of the posttrauma environment have received little attention but may be equally important. For example, in the case of Vietnam veterans, the attitude of society toward the war and the suddenness with which soldiers returned to the United States often created a hostile recovery environment. In his study of Canadian Vietnam veterans, Stretch (1990) suggests that the lack of societal recognition and the isolation from other veterans may have been even more damaging than the hostile or negative societal reaction in the United States.

Although there seems to be little data on the relationship between characteristics of the traumatic incident and the type or severity of symptomatic response, more systematic hypotheses are beginning to appear. Wilson et al. (1985) propose relationships between stressor dimensions, such as duration of trauma, severity of threat and loss, potential for recurrence, and the role of the person in the trauma, with particular P.T.S.D. symptomatology.

Attention to unique group differences in symptomatology can aid in the conceptualization of this disorder. In our investigation of injured workers with P.T.S.D. following traumatic work accidents (Howes & Parrott, in review), we found several striking features apparently more characteristic of this group than others described in the literature. As illustrated in Table 1, multiple forms of reexperiencing were frequently displayed (i.e., nightmares, ruminations, and flashbacks) by our patients. This presentation differs from other groups described in the literature, where one form of reexperiencing may predominate the clinical picture. For example, recurrent nightmares have been found to characterize P.T.S.D. following combat exposure (Brett & Ostroff, 1985), while Madakasira and O'Brien (1987) found that this particular symptom was infrequent in a sample of victims of a natural disaster who developed P.T.S.D. In an information-processing conceptualization of P.T.S.D., reexperiencing phenomena may be viewed as cued memory reactivation. Exposure to a greater number of retrieval cues might be expected for injured workers than for victims (who were not physically injured) of a natural disaster, since pain was a major problem for almost all of our patients and can be seen as a persisting internal retrieval cue. Generalized anxiety, phobic anxiety, and depressive features were also characteristic of our injured worker group (Table 1), whereas anger and guilt were less characteristic. This contrasts with past research in which anger, interpersonal difficulties, and hypervigilance have been identified as central symptoms displayed by Vietnam veterans with P.T.S.D. and survivor guilt in some concentration camp survivors (Daniele, 1985; Keane et al., 1985a). These observed differences in symptomatology may

TABLE 1. Frequency of Selected P.T.S.D. Symptoms
Reported by a Group of 53 Injured Workers
Diagnosed with P.T.S.D.[a]

| Symptoms[b] | Frequency | % |
|---|---|---|
| Reexperiencing phenomena | | |
|    Nightmares | 52 | 98 |
|    Ruminations | 41 | 77 |
|    Flashbacks | 34 | 64 |
| Phobic anxiety | 48 | 91 |
| Generalized anxiety | 42 | 79 |
| Depressed mood | 44 | 83 |
| Anger | 28 | 53 |
| Aggressiveness | 4 | 8 |
| Guilt | 3 | 6 |
| Pain complaints | 52 | 98 |
| Pretrauma psychological problems[c] | 10 | 19 |

[a] These data are taken from a larger descriptive study conducted by Howes & Parrott (in review).
[b] Symptoms listed in order of relevance to the diagnosis of P.T.S.D.
[c] Defined by a history of psychological treatment.

have implications for therapy and resolution of specific posttraumatic stress disorders. What is needed at this time is a systematic comparison, within a single study, of different P.T.S.D. groups.

## COGNITIVE ASSESSMENT ISSUES

The subjective experience of a traumatic event has received limited attention in the literature but has implications for cognitive assessment. The relevance of an individual's phenomenology is clear for the emotional disorders (Beck, 1976; Beck & Emery, 1985; Beck, Rush, Shaw, & Emery, 1979), and we argue that the same is true for P.T.S.D. The cognitive experience of the posttraumatic stress disorder victim has generally been dealt with in a descriptive manner, identifying characteristic symptoms (e.g., survivor guilt). However, descriptive approaches do not accurately represent the importance of cognitions (content, process, structure) in influencing distress and guiding coping. We propose that there are four cognitive issues which are particularly important to address within the P.T.S.D. population. Detailed evaluation of these issues can form the basis of a cognitive assessment. The information generated by such an assessment can be used to develop a treatment conceptualization.

## Appraisal of Trauma

Although in DSM-III-R a traumatic event is defined as "outside the range of usual human experience" (p. 247), we suggest that the victim's appraisal of the event is central to whether the event is traumatizing. The difficulty with the DSM-III-R criterion can be appreciated in a situation where the accident may be regarded as within the range of usual human experience, but a P.T.S.D. does develop (e.g., a minor motor vehicle accident where there has been no external life threat). This prob- lem can also be appreciated in situations where there is disagreement among mental health professionals concerning whether a specific event is within or outside usual human experience. The following case example illustrates this difficulty and emphasizes the role of one's appraisal of the trauma (both the victim's and the clinician's appraisal).

> This 50-year-old worker was involved in a verbal altercation with her supervisor. She became upset and subsequently began to panic and hyperventilate. Neither she nor her co-workers recognized what was happening. An ambulance arrived, and oxygen was administered, but the valve was not properly opened. The patient continued to have difficulty breathing and thought she was going to die. She was admitted to hospital and underwent medical investigations. No organic cause was identified for her breathing problems, and it was concluded she had hyperventilated. Despite the absence of an actual life-threatening accident or trauma, and despite medical reassurances, this patient developed a P.T.S.D. with recurrent nightmares, intrusive recollections, and generalized anxiety and depressive features. In this case, the development of P.T.S.D. appeared to be related to her cognitive appraisal of the events surrounding her breathing difficulties and her conclusion that her life was in danger.

In assessing an individual's appraisal of a traumatic event, it is also important to attend to selective perception and recall. A selective focus on the most vulnerable aspects of an incident may increase the traumatizing impact, while instrumental or survival behavior may be ignored.

## Generalized Belief of Vulnerability

As stated by Janoff-Bulman (1985), most of us operate under an assumption of invulnerability, a fundamental belief that the world is controllable and safe. This assumption is adaptive in that it protects us from the stress of contemplating all the possible misfortunes that might befall us. Janoff-Bulman (1985) postulates that the belief of invulnerability is "challenged by the experience of victimization" (p. 18). This assumption of invulnerability is "shattered" in patients with P.T.S.D. An overpowering and pervasive sense of vulnerability is experienced, characterized by heightened awareness of environmental threats (vigilance) and anticipation of future uncontrollable disasters (catastrophizing). In many cases this heightened belief of vulnerability can be seen as a central or core belief (see Safran, Vallis, Segal, & Shaw, 1986), which has significant impact on the individual's daily functioning.

This sense of vulnerability is most strongly associated with the traumatic event (learned alarm). However, we found in our study of injured workers (Howes & Parrott, in review) that stimuli which were not symbolic of, or similar to, the traumatic event could also trigger anxiety reactions. For instance, phobic anxiety toward driving an automobile frequently occurs. Excessive concern for the safety of others may also develop. The perception of vulnerability to possible threat or danger is consistent with Beck's conceptualization of anxiety disorders in terms of the cognitive sets of danger and vulnerability (Beck & Emery, 1985).

The following case highlights an example of a core belief of vulnerability and generalization of phobic anxiety, as well as the significance of subjective appraisal of the trauma.

> This 46-year-old factory worker sustained lacerations to her dominant arm and fractures of two fingers, when they became caught in a conveyor belt. She recovered almost full use, strength, and mobility of her hand and arm. Although the injury was not of a severe nature, her appraisal of the accident at the time was traumatizing. She had images of her arm being dragged into the machine and amputated by being pulled from the socket. She displayed classic P.T.S.D. symptoms and demonstrated a phobic response to the accident machine and the work place. In addition, phobic anxiety and avoidance generalized to household appliances including the electric blender, sewing machine, and iron, as well as to driving an automobile. She developed an overprotective attitude toward her three children (e.g., she cancelled their social activities that took them out of her sight). She also developed a preoccupation with her medical health as well as that of her family, and catastrophized about terrible illness and injury befalling them all.

In this case, one can readily appreciate the degree of impairment associated with these symptoms, based on this woman's generalized belief of personal vulnerability.

## Self-Questioning

Survivors of a traumatic event often become preoccupied with trying to establish some explanation and meaning, or cause, for their experience. This can be adaptive in terms of processing and integrating their experience, depending on the attributions made. Examples of adaptive attributions are: (1) an appropriate external, modifiable cause, as in the case of an industrial accident where a mechanical safety device malfunctioned, and/or (2) an internal, modifiable cause, such as attributing the accident to some aspect of one's behavior which would allow for increased control in the future by changing behavior (e.g., failure to check the safety device prior to using an industrial machine).

Maladaptive attributions can develop and often lead to the maintenance of P.T.S.D. symptoms. This may be more problematic in situations where the factors responsible for the traumatic event are not readily identifiable. Some survivors believe that they have little or no control over the trauma and develop maladaptive external attributions which lead to depression, isolation, and fear of recurrence (i.e., learned helplessness; Seligman, 1975; Seligman & Garber, 1980). This idea is partially supported by Mikulincer and Solomon (1988), who studied Israeli soldiers with combat stress reactions. They found that P.T.S.D. symptomatology was associated with a general attribution of both good and bad events to external and uncontrollable causes.

Some individuals may also view their tragic experience as punishment for past transgressions. Similarly, the "just world hypothesis" (Lerner, 1980), which suggests that victims are often perceived as responsible for their own adversity, may contribute to a critical self-perception. This type of characterological self-attribution may occur even when the cause of the accident or event is obviously external. Alternatively, an employer/co-worker, in the case of an industrial accident, or another external agent, may be viewed as culpable, regardless of his/her actual role. This type of attribution may lead to anger, bitterness, and often litigious behavior. Fifty-three percent of our injured worker sample reported problems with anger.

The type and adaptiveness of the attributions may vary between victims of natural disasters and man-made disasters and be affected by whether others have shared the same fate. An act of God which affects a large segment of the community would be expected to have a different impact than an intentional, malicious action toward an individual (Wilson et al., 1985). In the latter situation, a sense of vulnerability may be heightened by the possibility of further incidence or recurrence, and anger may be more clearly directed at the source.

## Self-Appraisal

The victimization experience and its aftermath can have a devastating impact on an individual's self-appraisal (Janoff-Bulman, 1985). As previously discussed, a characterological negative attribution for the occurrence of the traumatic event can be integrated into one's self-image. Attributing the cause of an accident to being a "stupid person" would be more damaging to self-esteem than a behavioral attribution that one had made a mistake. The experience of traumatic stress symptoms can also result in negative self-appraisal. Intrusive recollections, nightmares, intense fears, anxiety attacks, and emotional lability are frightening and ego-dystonic experiences which often prompt self-appraisals of weakness, helplessness, and loss of control. The fear of posttraumatic stress symptoms can itself become disabling and overwhelming. Frequently, this type of self-derogation prevents the individual from communicating his/her tumultuous feelings to others. Nadler and Ben-Shushan (1989) found that male Holocaust survivors were more poorly adjusted than female survivors. They noted that for males the experience of helplessness may be more incongruent with their self-perception and, as such, might partially account for this difference.

In an analog study with healthy undergraduates, Pennebaker and Beall (1986) suggested that failure to disclose about traumatic incidents may result in an increase in stress-related problems. They demonstrated that ventilation through essay writing was associated with fewer medical problems in a six-month follow-up period, as measured by health center visits. By failing to disclose, the individual with P.T.S.D. is not only depriving himself/herself of support and treatment, but his/her withdrawal may contribute to negative evaluation from significant others. Due to limited understanding of the victim's experience, significant others can contribute to his/her sense of alienation and negative self-image by denying the seriousness of the traumatic event. Alternatively, significant others may intentionally avoid contact with individuals suffering from P.T.S.D. due to their irritable, anxious, and fearful behavior. This process is akin to the interpersonal pattern seen in depression (Coyne, 1976).

Unfortunately, health care professionals may also contribute to an individual's low self-esteem and negative self-appraisal. The general practitioner is often the individual's first contact in the health system. If this professional has a limited understanding of P.T.S.D., an inaccurate diagnosis may be made. Consequently, the treatment recommended is likely to be unsuccessful and reinforce a sense of failure, helplessness, and hopelessness. Somatic complaints associated with a P.T.S.D. may divert treatment to multiple medical investigations and medication trials. The mental health professional providing therapy must also be aware of his/her own response to details of the traumatic event. Gruesome details may elicit a horrified or avoidance response on the part of the therapist, reinforcing the victim's belief that the trauma is too terrible to talk about. There may be moral principles involved with the individual's actions during the traumatic event (e.g., the rape victim who decides not to fight an armed attacker), which could elicit a judgmental response, again reinforcing a negative self-evaluation. Dealing with victims of traumatic experiences can challenge a therapist's own belief system and sense of meaning. The importance and value of the therapeutic relationship will be discussed in more detail later in this chapter.

## Cognitive Therapy for P.T.S.D.

There is little research into the efficacy of psychological treatments for P.T.S.D. However, some success has been reported using implosive techniques and relaxation training. For example, Hickling, Sison, and Vanderploeg (1986) examined the use of relaxation training and biofeedback on six patients with P.T.S.D. and reported slight to marked improvement for each patient. Keane and Kaloupek (1982) used relaxation and imaginal flooding in the treatment of a 36-year-old Vietnam veteran with P.T.S.D., and they reported a significant reduction in P.T.S.D. symptoms at 12-month follow-up. Recent research by Keane, Fairbank, Caddell, and Zimering (1989), in which implosive therapy was used with 24 veterans, supports the value of this technique in the treatment of P.T.S.D. Other researchers have found implosive and fantasy desensitization helpful following rape trauma (Rychtarik, Silverman, VanLandingham, & Prue, 1984) and motor vehicle accidents (McCaffrey & Fairbank, 1985). Grigsby (1987), on the other hand, used implosive imagery in conjunction with psychodynamic psychotherapy (i.e., abreaction and working through), but without relaxation, to treat a Vietnam veteran and reported decreased frequency of posttraumatic intrusive recollections. Collectively, these studies suggest that behavioral treatment is useful. A major difficulty, however, is that P.T.S.D. symptoms are often resistant to extinction. The reasons for lack of extinction are multifaceted and include avoidance of aversive memories; negative reinforcement of competing emotions such as anger; affective state dependent storage of memories, where access to the complete traumatic event is limited by physiological arousal (Keane *et al.*, 1985a); and continuous reminders of the trauma. Continuous reminders might include chronic pain from an injury or environmental cues which cannot be avoided. In the injured worker population, chronic pain not only stimulates and triggers recall of the accident, but it can also elicit kinesthetic imagery of the original injury. In this particular patient population, anticipatory anxiety associated with returning to the same or similar work environment can also have a profound impact.

While behavioral techniques are useful, it is our belief that cognitive therapy is well suited to this population. We recommend that initially the individual be assessed from a cognitive perspective to understand his/her appraisal and evaluation of the trauma, his/her generalized belief of vulnerability and how this belief has impacted on his/her functioning, his/her attributions and explanations concerning the trauma, and the resultant self-appraisal. At a conceptual level, we propose that these four components interact and affect both the victim's ability to function as well as their symptomatology. Examples of questions that facilitate exploration of these cognitive issues include the following: "What were you thinking and feeling at the time of the trauma and directly following?" "When you question why the trauma happened, what reasons come to mind?" "What are you fearful of since the trauma?" "How has your experience changed you?" and "Tell me about the activities you did and enjoyed before the trauma and what you do now?" The use of imagery and role play to aid in the recall of relevant cognitions at the time of the trauma is often helpful (see Beck *et al.*, 1979, for further details on the use of imagery and role play for assessing cognitions). Having the patient use thought records to prospectively collect negative cognitions is also recommended. Using responses to these probes, one can then develop a cognitive conceptualization of the patient's difficulties, which can be used to guide treatment.

In working with the P.T.S.D. population, there are several issues central to the implementation of cognitive therapy. First, given the factors involved in the formation and maintenance of P.T.S.D., the patient's presenting symptoms, and the patient's psychological insight and preexisting personality features, flexibility in treatment is necessary. Second, knowledge and appreciation of mediating factors such as cultural or religious beliefs that influence how the trauma is processed is important in conceptualization. Third, the development of a strong therapeutic relationship provides a safe context for the P.T.S.D. victim, which is often necessary when dealing with highly emotionally charged material. Fourth, acknowledgment of the impact of the trauma is useful in conceptualization, as well as treatment. Fifth, working with, rather than against, the "resistance" displayed by patients can be fruitful when treating P.T.S.D. victims (see Chapter 3, this volume). Finally, early recognition and intervention appears to be important and may prevent chronic disorders. Each of these treatment issues will be discussed in further detail in the remainder of the chapter. Case examples are presented to illustrate these points. Implementation of standard cognitive therapy interventions (e.g., rational responding, conducting behavioral experiments) will not be highlighted, as these techniques are familiar to cognitive therapists, and numerous texts are available that illustrate these techniques (e.g., Beck & Emery, 1985; Beck et al., 1979). The focus of this section is to examine the issues unique to cognitive therapy with P.T.S.D.

## Flexibility

In the therapeutic process, the selection and timing of interventions is critical. For example, if the therapist moves too quickly into implosive techniques, he/she may risk losing the patient who is not yet able to tolerate this, emotionally or cognitively. On the other hand, moving too slowly into implosive techniques may disillusion some patients, by suggesting to them that the *therapist* is unable to cope with the trauma. In some situations, it may be appropriate to provide more structure early in therapy (e.g., structured relaxation training) to increase the patient's sense of control and provide immediate symptom relief. Alternatively, structured interventions may be less successful in the early stages of therapy in some cases because a strong therapeutic relationship has not yet been established. Relaxation training, for example, may be rejected due to fear of further loss of control. Similarly, the selection and timing of cognitive techniques must be approached in a flexible manner.

Hyperarousal and a high basal level of anxiety are common symptoms of P.T.S.D. Individuals with P.T.S.D. often report a complete loss of control. This high level of anxiety can interfere with the patient's ability to concentrate, and this often interferes with cognitive interventions. Focusing on catastrophic cognitions or core issues of vulnerability initially may increase anxiety to an overwhelming level. In this situation, the therapeutic direction might be to strengthen the patient's sense of control. This can be done with distancing techniques such as projecting images on a television screen or using guided imagery where the therapist strongly emphasizes that this is a journey in imagination (e.g., the therapist often states, "no matter how real, you're in control, I'm with you"). As well, education about what to expect helps to increase the individual's sense of control.

In implementing cognitive therapy with P.T.S.D., the therapist must constantly attend to the therapeutic alliance, maintaining a trusting and safe environment in which to validate the patient's experiences. Feedback from the patient regarding the process of treatment assists in decision-making about implementation of treatment techniques. Further, we recommend a trial intervention method to help guide therapists to select an appropriate focus. By introducing an intervention, examining its initial efficacy, and carefully assessing the patient's reaction to the intervention, the therapist can make decisions about useful therapeutic strategies.

The following cases illustrate the importance of flexibility in cognitive therapy with P.T.S.D. and highlight the use of specific cognitive and behavioral strategies. In the first case, the aggravation of P.T.S.D. by a personal stressor unrelated to the trauma is illustrated. The patient's readiness for treatment was of primary importance in selecting therapeutic techniques.

*Case A*

> Mrs. A was a 35-year-old factory worker who was injured when her hair became caught in the fan of a cutting machine, and a large piece of scalp was torn from the left side of her head. The fact that another worker died following a head injury a few weeks earlier contributed to her trauma and her view that her injury was life threatening. She was diagnosed with P.T.S.D. and displayed the following symptoms: vivid recall of the accident, frequent nightmares and flashbacks, diminished interest in activities, anxiety symptoms, memory difficulties, tension-related headaches, and excessive somatic concern. This patient was initially seen in therapy for approximately four months one year following the accident. At that time, therapy focused on cognitive and behavioral coping skills to deal with specific and generalized anxiety symptoms. The use of coping self-statements, relaxation strategies, and distraction techniques were helpful. A strong therapeutic alliance was useful in providing a safe environment and facilitating the mobilization of coping resources. Considerable improvement occurred. However, a few months following the end of treatment, she had a frightening miscarriage and did not receive prompt medical care. She was away from home at this time and had limited support available. This personal trauma reinforced her core belief of vulnerability and significantly aggravated her P.T.S.D. symptoms related to her traumatic work accident. When she was seen in therapy again a few months later (for approximately eight months), she was having great difficulty functioning on a daily basis, and her anxiety had generalized to other situations (e.g., driving an automobile).

When seen for the second time, treatment proceeded as follows. Imagery strategies were used to decatastrophize (Beck & Emery, 1985) negative thoughts and images related to the work place, but these were only partially successful. Mrs. A had difficulty controlling her images of the cutting machine, because they elicited her memory of the accident and resulted in intolerable anxiety, which she was unwilling to endure. There was no significant evidence of extinction over repeated imaginal exposures. It became clear that she was not ready to deal with the intense anxiety and memory of the trauma directly, and thus, this approach was terminated. Contrary to Keane's (1988) general suggestion, rapid movement into exposure-based techniques does not appear to be helpful for all patients. Instead, therapy focused on problem solving and cognitive restructuring, targeting catastrophic cognitions following her nightmares (i.e., "I am going to die"; "I am going crazy"), as well as anxiety-related cognitions (e.g., "I am afraid I'll be reinjured"; "I can't cope"). Catastrophic and negative cognitions about her current situation, her ability to cope, and the future were central to her ongoing P.T.S.D. symptoms. Standard cognitive therapy techniques developed by Beck and his colleagues (Beck & Emery, 1985) were employed to deal with catastrophic and negative cognitions (i.e., identifying negative thoughts, challenging her thoughts, focusing on alternative interpretations, developing coping thoughts). Crisis management was employed to deal with an anniversary reaction (i.e., intensification of P.T.S.D. symptoms around the anniversary of her accident; anniversary dates are a common trigger of P.T.S.D. symptoms). Mrs. A responded positively to treatment, and by the end of therapy she was experiencing fewer nightmares, had increased her activity level, and was driving again. She subsequently gave birth to a healthy baby several months later.

The second case is an example of a severe, chronic P.T.S.D. Preexisting traumas appeared to contribute to the development of this man's stress disorder. Again, flexibility was essential in treatment.

## Case B

Mr. B was a 51-year-old roofer, who had worked in the construction industry for 30 years. He was injured when he fell 20 feet from a steep roof and sustained a minor head injury. Prior to this accident, he had fallen on three occasions and sustained significant injuries in one fall 10 years earlier. In the past, he returned to work on all occasions. It is noteworthy that a close family member committed suicide approximately 15 years earlier. When this man was seen two years after the last accident, P.T.S.D. and a major depressive episode were diagnosed. His symptoms included: frequent traumatic nightmares (i.e., falling off a roof), phobic anxiety to heights and generalization to other activities, generalized anxiety features, withdrawal and depressed mood, occasional suicidal ideation, severe tension-related headaches, and an intense belief of vulnerability. For example, he would walk on people's lawns rather than on the sidewalk, because he was fearful a car would leave the road and hit him. Clearly, he was functionally impaired.

A more unstructured, process-focused cognitive therapy approach was employed with this man, given the chronicity and severity of his symptoms, as well as the intensity of his core belief of vulnerability. He was seen for therapy over a one-and-a-half-year period. The initial focus was on the development of a strong therapeutic alliance and support. This resulted in a safe environment for him to explore his difficulties and to question his generalized belief of vulnerability. Relaxation training was employed to cope with headaches, generalized anxiety, and the aftermath of frightening nightmares. He developed an increased sense of self-efficacy in these areas. Distraction and increasing his activity level, as well as increasing social supports, were helpful in terms of depressive features. The development of these coping strategies was used by the therapist to help Mr. B reappraise his belief that he could not cope. Cognitive restructuring exercises (i.e., challenging dysfunctional thoughts) and coping self-statements were useful in helping him deal with depressive and anxious thoughts which tended to exacerbate emotional difficulties (e.g., "I can't cope"; "I can't relax"; "Everything is hopeless"; "I'm so anxious"). Crisis management and problem solving focused primarily on helping him cope with increased suicidal ideation and depressive features when his headaches were intense. Throughout therapy, Mr. B was also taking antidepressant and anxiolytic medication, which were prescribed and monitored by a psychiatrist. No attempt was made to address his catastrophic thoughts and fear of roofing through imaginal techniques, because he adamantly stated he would never return to this type of work. However, he did confront some aspects of the memory of his trauma imaginally. By the end of treatment he continued to display posttraumatic stress disorder symptoms and depressive features, but the frequency and intensity of these symptoms had decreased. He was using social supports more effectively and he continued in psychiatric treatment.

## Mediating Factors

The previous case histories illustrate potential mediating factors in the development and maintenance of P.T.S.D. that have received little attention; specifically, pre- and posttrauma stressors. These may be of a traumatic nature, such as a death, or less severe stressors, such as marital disharmony. Green, Wilson, and Lindy (1985) suggest that prior exposure to traumatic incidents may increase vulnerability. In our study of injured workers with P.T.S.D. (Howes & Parrott, in review), 36% of the sample had experienced a significant pretrauma stressor (e.g., death of a family member, previous accident and injury). The first case described above, Mrs. A, illustrates how subsequent stressors may aggravate or reactivate P.T.S.D. symptoms. Mrs. A integrated elements of the personal stress (i.e., miscarriage) into the P.T.S.D. nightmares. In the second case, pretrauma stressors likely served to increase Mr. B's vulnerability. That is, Mr. B may have been more vulnerable to developing P.T.S.D. due to past family tragedies and past accidents at work.

The *chronicity* of P.T.S.D. is now being appreciated in current research with Vietnam veterans, who continue to manifest symptoms for years following the onset of the disorder. Keane (1988) considers P.T.S.D. to be a lifelong disorder, at least in the population of veterans he works with. He identifies numbing of responsiveness as the core of the disorder and symptoms such as flashbacks and intrusive recollections as phasic, aggravated by life stressors. Thus, as illustrated in Case A, it may not be reasonable to expect a severe P.T.S.D. to resolve completely, but perhaps to be only deactivated. A further example of this is the case of a 44-year-old factory worker who was a Vietnam veteran. An industrial accident and persisting medical problems were the life stressors which reactivated combat-related P.T.S.D. symptoms from traumatic experiences 18 years earlier. Without an understanding of this patient's combat history, his hair-trigger rage response, nightmares, and episodes of depersonalization would seem a bizarre or even psychotic condition.

Green and Berlin (1987) provide empirical support for the significance of current life stress in P.T.S.D. In a study of psychosocial variables associated with P.T.S.D., current level of life stress was one of the five variables identified in a discriminant analysis. Life stress together with combat intensity correctly classified 75% of the cases. Further, Davidson and Baum (1986) report results indicating that mild symptoms of P.T.S.D. can occur following exposure to chronic stress (i.e., related to the Three Mile Island nuclear accident in 1979). These findings emphasize that the role of chronic life stressors should not be underestimated.

The mediating factors of pre- and posttrauma stressors are integral to conceptualizing cognitive issues. When an individual is attempting to integrate or find meaning in a traumatic experience, other significant experiences may influence the processing of the event. Previous exposure to a trauma could provide evidence that the world really is threatening, unsafe, and uncontrollable. The content of catastrophic cognitions may only be comprehensible in the context of the mediating stressful experiences.

## Therapeutic Relationship

As illustrated in the previous case examples, an atmosphere of safety and trust can be used to facilitate a reappraisal of the self as vulnerable. In addition, the therapist needs to validate the patient's experience by listening to any information offered without censor. Self-disclosure, as previously mentioned, may be uncomfortable for some patients due to negative self-appraisal, guilt, shame, or fear of being judged. Suspiciousness and mistrust are often symptomatic and can be dealt with through the therapeutic alliance.

If a support system exists, one aim of therapy is to access this, perhaps by teaching the patient to communicate about his/her experience within the therapeutic relationship. Alternatively, the therapeutic relationship may be the individual's only supportive relationship, and the task then is to mobilize community supports. The sense of alienation and uniqueness common with this disorder can be alleviated by acceptance and support from others. A multidisciplinary team approach to treatment can be particularly valuable in this regard (e.g., social workers, occupational therapists). As noted previously, social support has frequently been identified in the literature as a significant moderating variable (Barlow, 1988; Barrett & Mizes, 1988; Green & Berlin, 1987).

The following case highlights the importance of the therapeutic relationship and the value of support and multidiscipline involvement.

This 38-year-old well-educated man was admitted to hospital during an episode of alcohol abuse with suicidal ideation. He had recently immigrated to Canada and was experiencing major adjustment problems. He displayed a posttraumatic stress disorder related to political imprisonment and torture in his native country and subsequent detention in a concentration camp in another country. During inpatient and then outpatient treatment, psychological treatment focused on developing a therapeutic alliance in which he felt safe to explore traumatic memories, acknowledgment of trauma, relaxation techniques, education about his emotional reaction, and cognitive restructuring and coping skills. Central dysfunctional cognitions included, "I can't cope," "I will never be normal," "I will always be sick." Challenging his dysfunctional thoughts and employing coping thoughts and alternative interpretations were helpful. Occupational therapy and social work involvement were especially helpful in developing social and community contacts and supports, as well as providing functional training in tasks such as cooking and grocery shopping to aid adjustment to life in Canada. This combined therapy approach resulted in significant reduction of posttraumatic nightmares and recollections and facilitated his adjustment.

## Acknowledgment of the Trauma

Acknowledgment of the impact of the trauma is a major strength of a cognitive therapy approach. Such acknowledgment is critical in developing a collaborative relationship with the patient, and it forms the basis for identifying the importance of cognitive factors in P.T.S.D. and its treatment. It may also be the case that acknowledgment might be a buffer against developing P.T.S.D. It is our subjective impression, within the context of work-related injuries, that P.T.S.D. symptoms may be less likely to occur following major amputations, where the accident and injury are clearly life threatening, than following nonamputation limb injuries. In more severe injuries (i.e., traumatic amputations), everyone involved clearly views the accident as traumatic. In less severe injuries, or in cases where amputation is not necessary, the patient may view the trauma as more serious than the family and treatment staff, and this discrepancy in perception may aggravate the P.T.S.D. (Howes & Parrott, in review). We hypothesize that this potential discrepancy may be largely due to acknowledgment and support. With the more serious injuries, there is consensus among treatment personnel, family and friends, and the victim when appraising the trauma and its consequences. Extensive emotional and physical support is provided from an early stage for the more severe physical injuries, which aids both psychological and physical rehabilitation. By assessing the degree of discrepancy between the patient's and significant others' perception of trauma, one can evaluate the impact of this on the development and maintenance of P.T.S.D. At the present time there is a need for empirical research to address this issue.

## Resistance

Resistance in the form of lack of motivation, ambivalence, or avoidance of therapeutic exposure may appear to occur in the early stages of treatment. Such resistance may be a self-protective process, and therapists should avoid blaming the patient for it (see Mahoney, 1988; Chapter 3, this volume). Fully reexperiencing the traumatic experience is an important step in the goal of integrating and accepting the experience and altering maladaptive cognitions and beliefs. However, overwhelming levels of anxiety that lead to avoidance, or extended denial, may be seen as a protection against the full impact of the experience. Attention to this process provides useful information to guide therapists in pacing therapy.

## Early Recognition and Treatment

Early identification of P.T.S.D. symptomatology and appropriate treatment in the acute phase may be useful in preventing the development of a chronic disorder. However, early identification can be difficult for the following reasons. First, P.T.S.D. may sometimes present an atypical clinical picture. For example, when somatization or physical injury and pain are present, attention may be directed away from psychological symptoms. Schottenfeld and Cullen (1986) have distinguished between typical and atypical P.T.S.D., where the latter involves reexperiencing of bodily states associated with the trauma rather than recollection of the trauma and/or emotional and bodily states. Second, numbing of responsiveness or persistent denial may not appear to be dysfunctional if not carefully assessed, or may be misdiagnosed as primary depression. Third, in a delayed P.T.S.D., or with reactivation of a previous P.T.S.D., the traumatic event may be temporally distant and consequently not receive appropriate attention from the patient and the therapist.

Assessment of an individual's cognitive processes, content, and structure can aid in differential diagnosis, as well as in therapy. Evaluation of cognitive issues such as the generalized belief of vulnerability and self-questioning may be helpful, for example, in differentiating P.T.S.D., with numbing of responsiveness as the primary symptom, from adjustment disorder, with depressed mood.

## CONCLUSIONS

In this chapter, we discussed the utility of a cognitive orientation in the diagnosis, conceptualization, and treatment of posttraumatic stress disorders. Attention to the subjective experience of the traumatic event is important to our understanding of the development and maintenance of this disorder. We highlighted four cognitive components when conducting a cognitive assessment and developing a treatment conceptualization. These four components are appraisal and evaluation of the traumatic experience, generalized belief of vulnerability, self-questioning (i.e., attributions and meaning), and self-appraisal. Although these issues seem to be common to traumatic stress disorders, they most likely vary according to individual factors and with characteristics of the traumatic event such as duration, degree of violation, and extent of loss. Variation may be reflected in different symptom presentation and chronicity of the disorder. Understanding common features, aided by the DSM-III classification of posttraumatic stress disorder, has advanced this area of study. However, empirical study of various P.T.S.D. groups and the factors which influence variability is necessary.

We recommend a cognitive-behavioral treatment orientation, recognizing the importance of targeting all levels of the anxiety response: stimulus cues, psychophysiological responses, and meaning (i.e., attributions, appraisals of event and self, core beliefs). Selection and timing of therapeutic techniques is guided by the cognitive conceptualization of this disorder, emphasizing the cognitive issues described above. Some of the treatment issues discussed in reference to posttraumatic stress disorder are characteristic of the approach highlighted throughout this book with nontraditional populations. Specifically, conceptualization of the disorder and its development, flexibility in the therapeutic process, and attending to the therapeutic relationship and the meaning of apparent resistance are key issues. More specific to posttraumatic stress disorder, we highlighted the importance of assessing mediating factors of pre- and posttrauma stressors. In addition, early recognition of traumatic stress symptoms and acknowledgment by care givers of the individual's trauma and suffering is essential for successful treatment. As the chronicity of posttraumatic stress disorder becomes increasingly recognized, the education of care givers with respect to this disorder becomes more important.

Further research examining the cognitive processing of traumatic events is needed. Clarifying the importance of subjective appraisal of an event as traumatic (e.g., life threatening) has diagnostic and therapeutic relevance. A significant discrepancy between self- and others' appraisal could result in misdiagnosis, if the DSM-III-R criterion defining a traumatic event as "outside the range of usual human experience" is adhered to stringently. In addition, a discrepancy would be expected to impact negatively on self-image and the recovery environment (e.g., early recognition and support). Traumatic stress reactions in response to cumulative exposures to the suffering and death of others (e.g., in the course of emergency service work) illustrates the difficulty of diagnosis when individual events are not appraised as traumatic. Treatment direction and cognitive issues may differ when an individual has been the victim of trauma as opposed to witnessing a tragic event.

In addition to studying the impact of a traumatic experience and the efficacy of therapeutic intervention, another important area for future research is prevention. This could involve assisting individuals who have a high potential for exposure to traumatizing situations (e.g., workers such as police officers, fire fighters, and emergency medical personnel who are routinely exposed to violence, death, and destruction) to prepare for and adjust adaptively to such events. A cognitive focus in this area might deal with adaptive appraisal and interpretation of events (e.g., assumptions of invulnerability, personal responsibility).

# References

American Psychiatric Association. (1980). *Diagnostic and statistical manual of mental disorders* (3rd ed.). Washington, DC: Author.

American Psychiatric Association. (1987). *Diagnostic and statistical manual of mental disorders* (3rd ed., rev.). Washington, DC: Author.

Barlow, D. H. (1988). *Anxiety and its disorders: The nature and treatment of anxiety and panic.* New York: Guilford.

Barrett, T., & Mizes, J. (1988). Combat level and social support in the development of post-traumatic stress disorder in Vietnam veterans. *Behavior Modification, 12,* 100-115.

Beck, A. T. (1976). *Cognitive therapy and the emotional disorders.* New York: International Universities Press.

Beck, A. T., & Emery, G. (1985). *Anxiety disorders and phobias: A cognitive perspective.* New York: Basic Books.

Beck, A. T., Rush, A. J., Shaw, B. F., & Emery, G. (1979). *Cognitive therapy of depression.* New York: Guilford.

Birkhimer, L. J., DeVance, C. L., & Muniz, C. E. (1985). Posttraumatic stress disorder: Characteristics and pharmacological response in the veteran population. *Comprehensive Psychiatry, 26,* 304-310.

Brett, E. A., & Ostroff, R. (1985). Imagery and post-traumatic stress disorder: An overview. *American Journal of Psychiatry, 142,* 417-424.

Coyne, J. C. (1976). Toward an international description of depression. *Psychiatry, 39,* 28-40.

Daniele, Y. (1985). The treatment and prevention of long-term effects and intergenerational transmission of victimization: A lesson from Holocaust survivors and their children. In C. R. Figley (Ed.), *Trauma and its wake: The study and treatment of post-traumatic stress disorder* (pp. 295-313). New York: Brunner/Mazel.

Davidson, L. M., & Baum, A. (1986). Chronic stress and posttraumatic stress disorders. *Journal of Consulting and Clinical Psychology, 54*(3), 303-308.

Foy, D. W., Sipprelle, R. C., Rueger, D. B., & Carroll, E. M. (1984). Etiology of post-traumatic stress disorder in Vietnam veterans: Analysis of preliminary, military, and combat exposure influences. *Journal of Consulting and Clinical Psychology, 52,* 79-87.

Green, M. A., & Berlin, M. A. (1987). Five psychosocial variables related to the existence of post-traumatic stress disorder symptoms. *Journal of Clinical Psychology, 43*(6), 643-649.

Green, B. L., Wilson, J. P., & Lindy, J. D. (1985). Conceptualizing post-traumatic stress disorder: A psychosocial framework. In C. R. Figley (Ed.), *Trauma and its wake: The study and treatment of post-traumatic stress disorder* (pp. 53-69). New York: Brunner/Mazel.

Grigsby, J. P. (1987). The use of imagery in the treatment of post-traumatic stress disorder. *The Journal of Nervous and Mental Disease, 175,* 55-59.

Helzer, J. E., Robins, L. N., & McEvoy, M. A. (1987). Posttraumatic stress disorder in the general population: Findings of the epidemiologic catchment area survey. *The New England Journal of Medicine, 317,* 1630-1634.

Hickling, E. J., Sison, G., & Vanderploeg, R. D. (1986). Treatment of post-traumatic stress disorder with relaxation and biofeedback training. *Biofeedback and Self-Regulation, 11,* 125-134.

Horowitz, M. (1986). *Stress response syndromes* (2nd ed.). NJ: Jason Aronson.

Howes, J. L., & Parrott, C. A. (in review). Post-traumatic stress disorder: A study of injured workers.

Hyer, L., O'Leary, W. C., Saucer, R. T., Blount, J., Harrison, W. R., & Boudewyns, P. A. (1986). Inpatient diagnosis of post-traumatic stress disorder. *Journal of Consulting and Clinical Psychology, 54,* 698-702.

Janoff-Bulman, R. (1985). The aftermath of victimization: Rebuilding shattered assumptions. In C. R. Figley (Ed.), *Trauma and its wake: The study and treatment of post-traumatic stress disorder* (pp. 15-35). New York: Brunner/Mazel.

Keane, T. M. (1988). *Trauma*. Workshop presented at Association for Advancement of Behavior Therapy Conference, New York.

Keane, T. M. (1989). Post-traumatic stress disorder: Current status and future directions. *Behavior Therapy, 20*, 149-153.

Keane, T. M., & Kaloupek, D. G. (1982). Imaginal flooding in the treatment of a post-traumatic stress disorder. *Journal of Consulting and Clinical Psychology, 50*, 138-140.

Keane, T. M., Fairbank, J. A., Caddell, J. M., Zimering, R. T., & Bender, M. E. (1985a). A behavioral approach to assessing and treating post-traumatic stress disorder in Vietnam veterans. In C. R. Figley (Ed.), *Trauma and its wake: The study and treatment of post-traumatic stress disorder* (pp. 257-294). New York: Bruner/Mazel.

Keane, T. M., Scott, W. O., Chavoya, G. A., Lamparski, D. M., & Fairbank, J. A. (1985). Social support in Vietnam veterans with post-traumatic stress disorder: A comparative analysis. *Journal of Consulting and Clinical Psychology, 53*, 95-102.

Keane, T. M., Fairbank, J. A., Caddell, J. M., & Zimering, R. T.(1989). Implosive (flooding) therapy reduces symptoms of PTSD in Vietnam combat veterans. *Behavior Therapy, 20*, 245-260.

Kilpatrick, D. G., Best, C. L., Veronen, L. J., Amick, A. E., Villeponteaux, L. A., & Russ, G. A. (1985). Mental health correlates of criminal victimization: A random community survey. *Journal of Consulting and Clinical Psychology, 53*, 866-873.

Krystal, J. H., Kosten, T. R., Southwick, S., Mason, J. W., Perry, B. D., & Giller, E. L. (1989). Neurobiological aspects of PTSD: Review of clinical and preclinical studies. *Behavior Therapy, 20*, 177-198.

Lerner, M. J. (1980). *The belief in a just world*. New York: Plenum.

Litz, B. T., & Keane, T. M. (1989). Information processing in anxiety disorders: Application to the understanding of post-traumatic stress disorder. *Clinical Psychology Review, 9*, 243-257.

Madakasira, S., & O'Brien, K. F. (1987). Acute post-traumatic stress disorder in victims of a natural disaster. *The Journal of Nervous and Mental Disease, 175*, 286-290.

Mahoney, M. J. (1988). The cognitive sciences and psychotherapy: Patterns in a developing relationship. In K. Dobson (Ed.), *Handbook of cognitive-behavioral therapies* (pp. 357-386). New York: Guilford.

Marks, I. M. (1987). *Fears, phobias, and rituals: Panic, anxiety and their disorders*. New York: Oxford University Press.

McCaffrey, R. J., & Fairbank, J. A. (1985). Behavioral assessment and treatment of accident-related PTSD: 2 case studies. *Behavior Therapy, 16*, 404-416.

McFarlane, A. (1988). The aetiology of post-traumatic stress disorder following a natural disaster. *British Journal of Psychiatry, 152*, 116-121.

Mikulincer, M., & Solomon, Z. (1988). Attributional style and combat-related post-traumatic stress disorder. *Journal of Abnormal Psychology, 97*, 308-313.

Nadler, A., & Ben-Shushan, D. (1989). Forty years later: Long-term consequences of massive traumatization as manifested by Holocaust survivors from the city and the Kibbutz. *Journal of Consulting and Clinical Psychology, 57*, 287-293.

Pennebaker, J., & Beall, S. (1986). Confronting a traumatic event: Toward an understanding of inhibition and disease. *Journal of Abnormal Psychology, 95*, 274-281.

Ryctarik, R. G., Silverman, W. K., VanLandingham, W. P., & Prue, D. M. (1984). Treatment of an incest victim with implosive therapy. *Behavior Therapy, 15*, 410-420.

Safran, J. D., Vallis, T. M., Segal, Z. V., & Shaw, B. F. (1986). Assessment of core cognitive processes in cognitive therapy. *Cognitive Therapy and Research, 10*, 509-526.

Schottenfeld, R. S., & Cullen, M. R. (1986). Recognition of occupation-induced post-traumatic stress disorder. *Journal of Occupational Medicine, 28*, 365-369.

Seligman, M. E. P. (1975). *Helplessness: On depression, development, and death*. San Francisco: W. H. Freeman.

Seligman, M. E. P., & Garber, J. (1980). *Human helplessness*. New York: Academic Press.

Solomon, Z. (1988). Somatic complaints, stress reaction, and post-traumatic stress disorder: A three-year follow-up study. *Behavioral Medicine, 14*, 179-185.

Stretch, R. H. (1985). Post-traumatic stress disorder among U.S. Army Reserve Vietnam and Vietnam-era veterans. *Journal of Consulting and Clinical Psychology, 53*, 935-936.

Stretch, R. H. (1986). Post-traumatic stress disorder among Vietnam and Vietnam-era veterans. In C. R. Figley (Ed.), *Trauma and its wake, Volume II: Traumatic stress theory, research, and intervention* (pp. 156-192). New York: Brunner/Mazel.

Stretch, R. H. (1990). Post-traumatic stress disorder and the Canadian Vietnam veteran. *Journal of Traumatic Stress, 3*, 239-254.

Stretch, R. H., Vail, J. D., & Maloney, J. D. (1985). Post-traumatic stress disorder among army nurse corps Vietnam veterans. *Journal of Consulting and Clinical Psychology, 53*, 704-708.

Thienes-Hontos, P., Watson, C. G., & Kucala, T. (1982). Stress-disorder symptoms in Vietnam and Korean War veterans. *Journal of Consulting and Clinical Psychology, 50*, 558-561.

Trimble, M. R. (1985). Post-traumatic stress disorder: History of a concept. In C. R. Figley (Ed.), *Trauma and its wake: The study and treatment of post-traumatic stress disorder* (pp. 5-14). New York: Brunner/Mazel.

Wilson, J. P., Smith, W. K., & Johnson, S. K. (1985). A comparative analysis of PTSD among various survivor groups. In C. R. Figley (Ed.), *Trauma and its wake: The study and treatment of post-traumatic stress disorder* (pp. 142-172). New York: Brunner/Mazel.

# 6

# The Application of Cognitive Therapy to Postpartum Depression

## MARK OLIOFF

## OVERVIEW

The identification of factors which contribute to postpartum depression has been the focus of a growing research literature (e.g., Cutrona & Troutman, 1986; O'Hara, 1986). In contrast, relatively little attention has been paid to issues involved in psychotherapy for postpartum depression. In the present chapter, a cognitive psychotherapy approach to working with postpartum depressed mothers is outlined. Recent innovations in the theory and practice of cognitive therapy (e.g., Guidano & Liotti, 1983, 1988; Safran, Vallis, Segal, & Shaw, 1986) allow for the development of a preliminary treatment model for postpartum depression. This model does not ignore the complexity of the phenomenon, allows for flexibility in intervention, and avoids the confusion which may arise from nontheoretically based eclecticism. In addition, the model proposed in this chapter can be adapted to prepartum interventions aimed at preventing the onset of postpartum depression. The present chapter begins with a discussion of the nature of postpartum depression and its clinical significance. This is followed by an explication of cognitive strategies for assessing risk, and for treatment/prevention of this important problem.

MARK OLIOFF • Department of Psychology, The Mississauga Hospital, Mississauga, Ontario L5B 1B8, Canada.

## THE NATURE OF POSTPARTUM DEPRESSION

Postpartum depression can be distinguished from the transient emotionality (i.e., the "maternity blues") reported by at least 50% of women during the first 10 days postpartum, and from the severe, but infrequent, affective psychoses experienced by 0.1% to 0.2% of new mothers (e.g., Hopkins, Marcus, & Campbell, 1984; Kendell, 1985). The term "postpartum depression" refers to a broad syndrome of non-psychotic depressive symptoms resembling depression in other populations (Hopkins *et al.*, 1984; Kendell, 1985; O'Hara, 1986). Approximately 10% to 20% of women experience postpartum depression of at least several weeks duration, and there are numerous case reports of depression persisting throughout the year after childbirth (Bridge, Little, Hayworth, Dewhurst, & Priest, 1985; Hopkins *et al.*, 1984; Pitt, 1968).

Despite symptom similarity, postpartum depression can be distinguished from major depression on cognitive criteria. In postpartum depression, the primary focus of the individual's phenomenology is on *perceived parenting self-efficacy, global self-appraisal of parenting ability,* and the *vulnerability of the infant.* The following scenario is prototypic of postpartum depression. The postpartum depressed woman characteristically is preoccupied with a belief that she is an inadequate mother (Pitt, 1968). The mother doubts her efficacy to carry out everyday parenting activities successfully and believes that she is failing her infant. The emotional valence of these cognitions can be magnified by perceptions of the infant as vulnerable to life-threatening, catastrophic events and by difficulties in discriminating everyday problems in infant care from more urgent concerns. As the depression progresses, global attributional processes (Abramson, Seligman, & Teasdale, 1978) function to broaden the cognitive focus from perceived failure in specific parenting behaviors (e.g., "I cannot soothe my infant when she is crying") to more general negative self-appraisals of one's basic capacity as a mother (e.g., "I am a bad mother"). Subsequent difficulties in rearing the infant are selectively attended to, magnified, and processed in a manner which is consistent with the woman's negative appraisals of her capacity to mother. As such, these appraisals become further entrenched.

The co-occurrence of beliefs that one is failing to parent adequately with perceptions of the infant as vulnerable to catastrophic events contributes to persistent agitation, anxiety, and apprehension about the baby's welfare (see Martin, 1977; Pitt, 1968). In addition, Olioff and Aboud (in press) report data which suggest that by the second month postpartum, negative self-appraisals about parenting have impacted on more general self-esteem. This suggests that the mother can become increasingly hopeless. Guilt is commonly experienced, stemming from the mother's feelings of frustration and deprivation, when she believes that she should be overjoyed with parenting. Further, social isolation is common, often associated with the mother's beliefs that her negative thoughts about parenting are socially unacceptable. Thus, potential opportunities for feedback which might challenge dysfunctional thinking are lost. In the more severe postpartum depressions, underlying developmental issues involving the mother's early experiences with her own parents and schemata regarding personal identity can be triggered, making the phenomenology of the depression more complex and idiosyncratic.

In summary, understanding postpartum depression is facilitated by attention to three overlapping cognitive features: (1) perceptions of the infant as vulnerable, (2) poor parenting self-efficacy, and (3) more global beliefs that one is an inadequate mother. In addition to the distress experienced by the depressed mother, these cognitive features may impede the development of adequate parenting skills. For instance, poor self-efficacy can contribute to a failure to master adequate coping behaviors by reducing effort and persistence in the face of obstacles to learning (e.g., Bandura, 1977, 1982; Cutrona & Troutman, 1986). This can be particularly destructive since flexible adaptation is required to parent throughout the child's rapid development (e.g., Grossman, Eichler, & Winickoff, 1980; Leifer, 1977). Even moderate levels of postpartum depressive symptoms in mothers may increase their infant's vulnerability to subsequent cognitive and behavioral problems during childhood (e.g., Cogill, Caplan, Alexandra, Robson, & Kumar, 1986; Uddenberg & Englesson, 1978; Wrate, Rooney, Thomas, & Cox, 1985). Moreover, postpartum depression appears to be associated with mothers' perceptions of marital discord and of deficits in spousal support (Kumar & Robson, 1984; O'Hara, 1986; O'Hara, Rehm, & Campbell, 1983; Paykel, Emms, Fletcher, & Rassaby, 1980). If these issues are not resolved, they can lead to longer-term disruptions in the relationship between parents (Grossman *et al.*, 1980; Kumar & Robson, 1984). Clearly, both infant and father, in addition to mother, can be affected negatively by postpartum depression.

## ASSESSING RISK FOR POSTPARTUM DEPRESSION

An exhaustive review of the research on factors which may increase vulnerability to postpartum depression is beyond the scope of the present chapter (see Hopkins *et al.*, 1984, and Kendell, 1985, for reviews).

However, the major findings are outlined with a focus on their clinical utility.

Several areas of research on potential risk factors have failed to yield significant results. There is no consistent evidence that any specific pregnancy- or delivery-related variable (e.g., complications, extent of planning, type of delivery) is predictive of postpartum depression. Similarly, characteristics of the expectant mother, such as her age, number of children, socioeconomic status, marital status, or religion, also are not reliable predictors (see Hopkins et al., 1984; Kendell, 1985). Physiological theories of postpartum depression have focused on endocrinological changes that occur during the early postpartum period (e.g., Dalton, 1980) and on neurochemical explanations (e.g., Handley, Dunn, Waldron, & Baker, 1980). As yet, there is no conclusive evidence that any physiological mechanism plays a significant causal role (e.g., Gelder, 1978; Hopkins et al., 1984; Youngs & Lucas, 1980).

The factors emerging from the research literature as predictors of postpartum depression are: (1) prepartum levels of depression (e.g., Atkinson & Rickel, 1984; O'Hara, Rehm, & Campbell, 1982), (2) life event stressors during pregnancy (e.g., O'Hara et al., 1982; Paykel et al., 1980), (3) poor social supports, particularly problems in the spousal relationship (e.g., O'Hara et al., 1983; Paykel et al., 1980), and (4) significant infant health risks and temperament problems (e.g., Blumberg, 1980; Cutrona & Troutman, 1986). The possible presence of each of these factors and the manner in which patients cope with them should be carefully evaluated in any clinical assessment of risk for postpartum depression. Preliminary evidence suggests that these factors may make distinct contributions to postpartum depression, such that the additional presence of each may increase risk (e.g., Cutrona & Troutman, 1986; O'Hara et al., 1982, 1983; Paykel et al., 1980). However, additional research is required to evaluate the complex interrelationships between these variables and the ways in which they may combine to contribute to postpartum depression.

## The Importance of Cognitive Appraisal

A basic tenet of cognitive therapy is that the manner in which individuals appraise their experiences is important in influencing affect and behavior (e.g., Beck, 1967; Ellis, 1962, 1980). This applies equally to postpartum depression. It is critical that the clinician assess each woman's view of her own pregnancy and parenting experience, including her appraisals of particular variables which may not have been shown to be risk factors in nomothetic research. For instance, many women adjust to unplanned pregnancies and do not evaluate their occurrence as reflecting upon their desire or ability to mother. However, a woman who believes that planning is an essential component of preparing for motherhood may experience an unplanned pregnancy as a significant failure. If this perceived failure generalizes to beliefs that she is failing as a mother, her vulnerability to depression during pregnancy and after childbirth may be increased.

Most of the available research on postpartum depression (including the multivariate studies) has focused on the main statistical effects of risk factors, rather than on specific interactions between them, or on the possible moderating role of cognitive appraisal mechanisms. The potential importance of cognitive mediation has recently been demonstrated by Cutrona and Troutman (1986). Using a multivariate path analysis, they found that perceived parenting self-efficacy moderated the impact of prepartum social supports and of infant temperament on postpartum depression. Thus, it may be important in clinical assessment to determine how a mother's perceived parenting self-efficacy is affected by major risk factors. For instance, a mother who is trying to raise a child with serious health risks or a difficult temperament may be more likely to have frustrating and difficult experiences. If these are appraised in a manner which contributes to poor parenting self-efficacy (e.g., attributing childrearing problems to personal inadequacy), the woman may be more at risk for postpartum depression.

Aside from a possible mediational role, there is some evidence from pre- to postpartum prospective studies to suggest cognitive vulnerability toward postpartum depression. Olioff and Aboud (in press) adapted Bandura's model of self-efficacy to evaluate pregnant women's expected parenting self-efficacy. They found that perceived parenting self-efficacy during the third trimester of pregnancy predicted intensity of dysphoria six weeks postpartum, after initial levels of dysphoria were statistically controlled. In similar prospective multivariate research, it has been shown that measures of prepartum attributional style (Abramson *et al.*, 1978) and of self-control attitudes (Rehm, 1977) are predictive of postpartum depressive symptoms (e.g., Cutrona, 1983; O'Hara *et al.*, 1982).

Thus, in line with clinical descriptions of the phenomenology of postpartum depression, there is some research to suggest that cognitive appraisal mechanisms may play significant mediational and/or predisposing roles in postpartum depression. While, as yet, there is no specific clinical outcome literature on cognitive therapy with the postpartum depressed, an extensive literature does exist on cognitive therapy for depression in the broader population (e.g., Beck, Rush, Shaw, & Emery, 1979). Guidelines for adapting cognitive therapy to the specific experiences of the postpartum depressed are discussed next.

## COGNITIVE THERAPY FOR POSTPARTUM DEPRESSION

In recent theoretical developments in cognitive therapy, the distinction between surface automatic thoughts (cognitive content) and underlying cognitive schemata (cognitive structure) has been elaborated (Guidano & Liotti, 1983, 1988; Safran et al., 1986). Associated with this, there has been increased specification of intervention strategies targeted at cognitive structure (see Guidano & Liotti's work on constructivist-based cognitive therapy). In line with these developments, one of the critical distinctions to be made in treating postpartum depression is whether to conceptualize contributing cognitive factors as problems in cognitive content or in underlying schemata. Treatment of cognitive content involves short-term, active efforts from the therapist to assist the patient in reappraising dysfunctional thoughts (e.g., Beck et al., 1979; Ellis, 1962, 1980). Treatment at the level of cognitive schemata, however, tends to involve a less structured, less didactic approach. More emphasis is placed on therapy process and the therapeutic relationship as means of identifying, and gradually restructuring, core cognitive processes (see Chapter 1, this volume). It should be noted that an empirically valid basis for distinguishing cognitive content from cognitive schemata awaits research. Nonetheless, this distinction is presently useful in developing a cohesive conceptual framework which facilitates selection of appropriate clinical intervention strategies. In the remainder of this chapter, guidelines for treatment of both of these therapeutic targets is outlined.

### Dysfunctional Cognitive Content

One of the interesting aspects of clinical work with the postpartum depressed is the number of patients who have a previous history of *good* psychological adjustment. Many women who seek help for postpartum depression have coped well with their lives in general and are experiencing their first depressive episode (Pitt, 1968; Kumar & Robson, 1984). Typically, these women are unprepared for the multifaceted changes involved in the transition to motherhood or, in the case of multiparous women, for the complex problems involved in integrating an additional child into the family (Grossman et al., 1980; Leifer, 1977). Moreover, dysfunctional beliefs that pregnancy and motherhood should be completely happy, stress-free periods pervade our culture and continue to influence the thinking of many mothers, so that they believe they are failing when problems do surface (Dix, 1985; Grossman et al., 1980). The most common cognitive problems these women display are at a content level, involving perceptions that their infants are vulnerable, perceptions of poor parenting self-efficacy, and more general appraisals that they are inadequate parents. *Unrealistic expectations* with respect to obstetrical matters, maternal attachment, and parenting performance contribute substantially to these cognitive content problems (see Table 1 for a description of typical dysfunctional expectations and associated automatic thoughts).

As outlined in Table 1, a unifying theme of many of the unrealistic expectations that postpartum depressed patients have about obstetrical matters is that a good mother should have a smooth biological transition to parenthood. A woman's recognition that she has failed to achieve these ideals may contribute to perceptions that she is an inadequate mother before she ever handles her child. Olioff and Aboud (in press) have shown that expectant, primiparous mothers already have developed perceptions of their parenting self-efficacy by the third trimester of pregnancy, perceptions which are significantly related to their postpartum appraisals of parenting self-efficacy.

Unrealistic expectations regarding maternal attachment dictate that good mothers only have positive feelings toward their infants (see Table 1). Postpartum depressed women often report guilt and remorse in having experienced frustration and irritation with their infants. Moreover, this often is interpreted as evidence that they are inadequate mothers.

TABLE 1. Dysfunctional Cognitions concerning Pregnancy and Parenthood

| Expectation | Related automatic thoughts |
|---|---|
| 1. The biological transition to parenthood should be smooth. | "My pregnancy and delivery should be free of complications." "I should not require use of anesthesia, forceps, or episeotomy." "I should have a vaginal delivery, not a caesarean." |
| 2. Attachment to the infant should be easy and free of negative feelings. | "I should always feel love for my baby." "Negative feelings toward my baby are wrong." |
| 3. Good mothers should have innate parenting abilities and have no legitimate personal needs. | "I should always know how to best care for my baby." "Childrearing should be natural, not difficult and frustrating." "I should always be available for my baby." "Now that I am a mother, my past lifestyle and activities should not be important." |

Finally, as documented in Table 1, misconceptions about parenting performance usually involve themes that good mothering is an innate quality of the mother, rather than a learned skill, and that a good mother's personal needs are of secondary importance. Postpartum depressed mothers often appraise everyday difficulties in childrearing as evidence of their inadequacy as parents (see Cutrona & Troutman, 1986). Attempts at self-gratification become associated with guilt and with thoughts that one is an inadequate mother. Failure to achieve parenting performance ideals increases anxiety that the infant is more vulnerable because he/she is not receiving adequate parenting.

The cognitions described above will be familiar to cognitive therapists on the basis of their rigid, extreme qualities and dysfunctional nature (Beck *et al.*, 1979; Ellis, 1962, 1980). As with cognitive distortions in major depression, processes such as magnification, generalization, and internal negative attributions (Abramson *et al.*, 1978; Beck *et al.*, 1979) operate to reinforce the emotional valence of these cognitions and thereby contribute to postpartum depression. Furthermore, it should be emphasized that the dysfunctional cognitions outlined in Table 1 are not exhaustive. The therapist must remain sensitive to the idiosyncratic appraisals of individual patients (Guidano & Liotti, 1983, 1988). In addition, he/she must be able to identify core (as opposed to peripheral) expectations that may account for consistent problems in appraisal of infant vulnerability, parenting self-efficacy, and broader parenting ability across a variety of perinatal experiences (see Safran *et al.*, 1986; Chapter 2, this volume).

In the following case description, criteria for determining that dysfunctional cognitions contribute to the onset or maintenance of a patient's postpartum depression are illustrated.

A 30-year-old female (D.W.) was referred for treatment of postpartum depression by her family physician. D.W. presented as an intelligent woman with a master's degree in business administration who was invested in a successful managerial career. Her marriage was in its eighth year. The couple had a five-year-old daughter in addition to their infant who was now seven weeks old. D.W. described her relationship with her husband as mutually supportive, noting that he encouraged her career endeavors and was actively involved in child care. The patient had additional social supports, including her mother, who had volunteered to assist with rearing the newborn. She had no previous contact with mental health professionals and no prior psychological problems. D.W. noted that there had been no additional stressors over the past year and that her infant was healthy. She emphasized that she had coped well with the birth of her first child and could not understand why she was feeling so depressed for the first time in her life.

In the initial session, D.W. reported feeling very guilty. She noted that she began to feel depressed on the day that she returned home from hospital and had been feeling increasingly depressed over the last month. Although she could not explain why, an early process marker of a potential core cognitive issue was the strong affect she exhibited when expressing thoughts about being unable to care for her infant. When asked to elaborate, D.W. disclosed that she thought of herself as an incompetent mother, and then became noticeably distraught. D.W. maintained this self-appraisal, although when asked to provide supporting evidence, she could only repeat that she was not being a good mother. When questioned directly, she acknowledged that she had not harmed the infant and was taking care of the infant's basic needs by relying on support from others. When this contradictory evidence was reflected back to D.W., she seemed embarrassed but also somewhat relieved.

When a postpartum depressed patient exhibits strong affect around cognitions of parenting self-efficacy, and evidence is obtained early in sessions that cognitive shifts can be made with consequent improvement in affect, the therapist should pursue the hypothesis that the primary dysfunction is in cognitive content (see Safran & Greenberg, 1986; Safran et al., 1986). Thus, in the second session the therapist focused increasingly on D.W.'s automatic thoughts regarding her inadequacy as a mother.

Horizontal exploration (Safran et al., 1986; see Chapter 2, this volume) revealed that D.W.'s negative parenting self-appraisals were associated with an awareness that she missed her job outside the home and disliked the current disruption in her lifestyle brought on by the newborn. D.W. admitted that she did not know if she could tolerate being at home for the four months maternity leave she had arranged because she missed the stimulation of other adults. She talked about how much she enjoyed her work, but acknowledged, "I could hold out until January." Her next automatic thoughts were "this is wrong," and "I feel bad." She timidly disclosed that she had not experienced any intense feelings of love for her infant and at times even felt irritated with her baby. When asked to elaborate further, D.W. broke down and cried, stating "I should be more devoted to my child" (again suggesting strong affect around parenting self-appraisals).

In the absence of other salient factors (life event stressors, social supports, infant characteristics, and prepartum affect did not appear problematic), it was hypothesized that the major factor contributing to D.W.'s postpartum depression was her excessive commitment to rigid, unrealistic ideals about maternal attachment and parenting performance. She appeared to be appraising her failure to achieve these ideals consistently as evidence that she was an inadequate mother. This in turn triggered feelings of guilt, despondency, and depression.

In arriving at a working conceptualization, the therapist should routinely assess the patient's historical relationship with her own mother. This is important because a woman's early experiences with her mother can contribute to her own beliefs about what is appropriate for the maternal role (e.g., Benedek, 1970). Moreover, evidence of a long-standing positive relationship with the patient's own mother suggests that misconceptions about parenting can be treated as dysfunctional cognitive content, as opposed to underlying schemata stemming from unresolved early parenting problems.

> In the third session, horizontal and vertical assessment were employed to reveal that D.W.'s maternal ideals were associated with her pleasant and possibly idealized memories of her own mother during her childhood. The patient noted that she had a happy childhood. She remembered that her mother did not work outside the home, "always was available," and seemed completely content to devote herself entirely to parenting. In this context, D.W. spontaneously revealed that she believed her mother had been "an ideal mother," that she believed she should be more like her mother, and believed it was wrong to have mixed feelings about her leave of absence to care for her children. When asked directly to evaluate herself as a mother in comparison with her own mother, D.W. described additional feelings of inadequacy.

Thus, evidence was obtained suggesting that D.W.'s beliefs about her & competence as a mother were based on unrealistic expectations associated in part with idealized memories of her own mother. D.W.'s awareness that she was failing to meet these expectations appeared to be triggering depression through internal negative attributions and self-blaming processes (Abramson et al., 1978; Beck, 1967; Beck et al., 1979).

To summarize, five criteria mark a case as one that can be conceptualized at the level of cognitive content: (1) the current episode is the patient's first depression, (2) the patient's previous psychological adjustment has been good, (3) there is a history of a positive childhood relationship with the patient's own mother, (4) strong affect is associated with the patient's negative parenting self-appraisals, and finally, (5) brief in-session cognitive interventions produce positive shifts in the patient's affect. If, in addition, there are no other major contributing factors (e.g., infant health risk, life event stressors, poor spousal support), the therapist can adopt a short-term treatment model. Such a model involves provision of educational information about the normative experience of mothers and active collaboration with the patient in challenging her dysfunctional thoughts. If the therapist is correct in conceptualizing that the major problems are in cognitive content, as opposed to underlying schemata, patient resistance to change should not be a significant factor. Improvement can usually be observed within 10 sessions. To return to our case:

Educational information was provided to D.W. regarding the difficulties many women now face in trying to balance parenting and career aspirations. She was reassured that her own conflicts in this area did not represent a failure to be a good mother. Rather, it was suggested that D.W. was expecting too much from herself in trying to live up to her idealized memories of her own mother, who had reared her in a different generation with different parenting values and socioeconomic circumstances. D.W. actively began to consider alternative models for parenting based on peers who combined motherhood with careers outside the home. She was encouraged to focus on her good adjustment and achievements with her first child, and on her current efforts to draw on additional supports in caring for her infant, as evidence that she was a good mother. She began to reappraise her internal negative attributions for "wrong feelings" toward her infant in light of information about how common such feelings actually are. The patient was encouraged to distinguish between feelings and performance, and to base her appraisal of her competence on the latter. She was given weekly homework assignments to help her focus on her positive achievements in child care. Gradually, she reported an increased number of child care behaviors and incidents which she appraised as evidence of competent parenting. Within seven weekly sessions, she was no longer reporting depression, was expressing renewed confidence in her capacity to parent, and no longer required her mother's assistance. In addition, she had become more accepting of her desire to return to work outside the home and no longer believed this meant that she was an inadequate mother. D.W. maintained her progress over the next month and sessions were terminated then at her request.

## Dysfunctional Cognitive Schemata

It has been hypothesized that women's constructs of motherhood and of themselves as mothers are shaped by their early experiences with their own mothers (e.g., Benedek, 1970; Keating & Manning, 1974). Moreover, there is some evidence that patients who have had conflicted relationships with their own mothers are more likely to have persistent conflicts about being mothers themselves, and may be vulnerable to postpartum depression (e.g., Heitler, 1976). In contrast to the relatively straightforward case of D.W. described above are those in which long-standing developmental issues involving the patient's relationship with her mother become exacerbated at the time of childbirth. Such cases are considerably more difficult to treat. Well-entrenched, underlying self-schemata regarding the affective meaning of motherhood exert a profound influence on how the patient appraises everyday issues involving parenting. In addition, these self-schemata become entangled with the patient's core constructs of self-worth. Unlike depressogenic automatic thoughts, such dysfunctional schemata are less directly accessible to the patient and often must be deduced by the therapist on the basis of therapy content and process. Moreover, as constructivist-based theorists have pointed out, cognitive schemata often are idiosyncratic, and tend to be resistant to change (e.g., Liotti, 1987; Safran et al., 1986). Therapeutic efficacy in such cases is contingent upon a model of treatment which facilitates exploration of the patient's schemata concerning motherhood, and the relationship of these schemata to core constructs of the self (see Guidano & Liotti, 1983, 1988; Safran et al., 1986).

To illustrate, let us consider a case in which themes of abandonment, related to recurrent experiences of loss and emotional rejection during childhood, dominated a patient's constructs of motherhood and profoundly shaped her appraisals of her parenting competence and self-worth. An unsuccessful attempt was made to treat this patient's depression at the level of cognitive content. The therapist was required to modify his approach in order to address underlying dysfunctional schemata.

A 31-year-old married female (N.K.), employed as a high school teacher, was seen initially during her fifth week postpartum complaining of increasing feelings of depression during the previous month. N.K. presented as an intelligent, articulate, first-time mother in a stable marital relationship. N.K. denied any significant disappointments about her pregnancy or delivery or any additional life event stressors during the previous year. She described her daughter as a healthy, pleasant baby and reported a strong affective bond with her.

N.K. noted that she began to feel discouraged during the second week postpartum because there were times when "I did not know what I should do when my daughter cried or appeared upset." She said this made her feel overwhelmed with the burden of responsibility of caring for her infant and that she was beginning to doubt her ability as a parent. She said that at times when she could not detect what her baby needed she had thoughts that "I am failing" and "I am a terrible mother." Her next automatic thoughts showed a link between these parenting appraisals and her more global notions of self-worth. The patient reported that "I had coped well with major challenges in my life in the past," and that not being able to care for her baby was the "worst thing that could happen in my life" and made her feel "like a failure." She stopped talking at this point in the session, in order to regain control of her emotions. This was the only time N.K. had exhibited strong affect in the session, which suggested the emotional significance of these parenting self-appraisals (Safran & Greenberg, 1986).

As there was no other apparent source of distress, and no history of prior emotional problems or contacts with mental health professionals, the initial focus of interventions was at the level of cognitive content regarding N.K.'s perceived parenting self-efficacy. In the second session:

> The therapist suggested that N.K. appeared to have high expectations for her performance as a parent and seemed to believe that being an effective, good mother meant that she should always know what to do with her infant. Comments such as these, as well as the provision of information about common parenting difficulties that new mothers experience, appeared to have the effect of making the patient feel more agitated. If anything, she increased her statements about her inadequacy as a parent and her lack of self-worth. Moreover, the therapist had the impression that N.K. appeared angry in the session and seemed to resent his efforts to offer support.

The failure of the therapist's efforts in the second session to impact on N.K.'s perceived parenting inefficacy and N.K.'s angry reaction to these efforts both suggested that it was inadequate to conceptualize her problem in terms of cognitive content. As such, in the third session, the therapist began to shift away from an actively supportive role involving the provision of education and collaborative challenging of automatic thoughts. A more nondirective stance was adopted with greater focus on the use of therapy process and the therapeutic relationship to explore for possible underlying dysfunctional schemata.

> After inquiring about N.K.'s experiences in the week between sessions, the therapist asked her how she felt about the sessions so far. N.K. was quiet and appeared uncomfortable. The therapist commented on this. When the patient did not respond again, he allowed for a greater lapse of silence. He then commented that the patient had appeared irritated or angry in the previous session and he asked how she was feeling now. N.K. seemed taken aback, but acknowledged that she had felt angry with the therapist in the previous session and, in the intervening week, had wondered about whether to continue with therapy. She could not explain why she felt angry, but added that she had never sought professional assistance before and that "Coming to see a psychologist made me feel weak and incompetent," "I was a strong person and this was not me." N.K. then appeared as though she was going to cry, but again, seemed to collect herself.
> The therapist again noted the strong affect N.K. exhibited when dis-

cussing her appraisals of competence. In addition, he began to speculate whether there was an underlying association for this patient between self-appraisals of inadequacy, feelings of anger, and possible conflicts around receiving support.

The above case illustrates the complex issues that the therapist may face in treating a postpartum depressed patient and the need for a flexible approach to treatment. When the therapist actively encouraged N.K. to challenge the content of her cognitions, she showed signs of anger and resistance. Indeed, one could speculate, based on N.K.'s report in the subsequent session, that had the therapist ignored these signs and continued actively encouraging N.K. to reevaluate her cognitive content, she might have withdrawn from therapy.

In addition to the modifications in conceptualization and approach discussed previously, it is important for the clinician to recognize that a patient's "resistance" may reflect the operation of stable underlying cognitive schemata, such as the tendency to screen out contradictory information, rather than motivational barriers at a dynamic level (see Liotti, 1987; Chapter 3, this volume). In this sense, resistance can be seen as a process marker of potential underlying cognitive schemata whose affective meaning needs to be assessed in a nondirective, nonthreatening manner which gradually encourages patient collaboration.

Further exploration, in the fourth session, of the possible association between appraisals of competence, anger, and conflicts regarding support revealed that N.K. had been experiencing strong, persistent resentment toward her mother since giving birth to her child, particularly when her mother offered to help with the infant's care. In this context, the patient remarked that she had an excellent relationship with her mother and was unaccustomed to experiencing persistent anger at her. Moreover, N.K. acknowledged that she had no reason to doubt that her mother could care for the infant, but still believed that she should be the one to do so. N.K. admitted that even having her mother babysit while she attended sessions provoked extreme anxiety and guilt. She added that although she usually trusted her husband, she avoided allowing him or anyone else to handle the baby whenever possible. At this point she became intensely agitated, and reported that she believed "I should not leave my baby for a moment." She reported that she was worried about her infant's vulnerability, and added that she was finding it difficult to sleep at night because she kept having intrusive thoughts that "something bad" was going to happen to her baby. Although N.K. could acknowledge that the baby was healthy and that "I am being irrational," she said "I do not care, I have to know that I always will be there for my baby."

Thus, more evidence was provided in the fourth session to suggest an association between N.K.'s parenting self-appraisals, her anger, and her reaction to the support of others, especially her mother. It appeared that for N.K. being a competent mother meant taking full responsibility for child care and, thus, offers of support from others provoked anger and had to be rejected. Perceptions of her infant's vulnerability appeared to magnify the affect attached to this patient's constructs of competent mothering.

Vertical assessment continued and involved an exploration of key developmental issues which may have contributed to the formation of N.K.'s cognitive schemata concerning parenting (see Safran *et al.*, 1986).

> In the sessions that followed, the therapist focused increasingly on exploring the meaning that N.K. attached to always being available for her child and why she perceived this as a critical basis for parenting competence. Over the course of eight months of sessions, it was revealed that the patient had a traumatic separation experience from her own mother during her second year of life. At the age of fourteen months, N.K.'s mother became severely ill and needed to be hospitalized for four months. For six weeks during this period, the patient had no contact with her mother whatsoever. Moreover, as her father was a businessman who was away from home for prolonged periods, the patient was taken in by her aunt who lived in another city. She had no siblings and, as such, the separation from her nuclear family was complete. Further, when the patient's mother returned home from hospital, she still was too ill to look after her child. N.K. pointedly noted that she had to stay on with her aunt for an extra two months.
>
> In the context of exploring these events, it gradually became evident that while N.K. idolized her mother in many respects, she had never felt that she could rely on her for emotional support during times of crisis. N.K. vividly recalled several subsequent experiences in her childhood and adolescence in which she had felt rejected by her mother when seeking support (e.g., when she was failing in a course at school). Over the years she developed the schema that competence required total emotional self-reliance. N.K. related how this had generalized to other relationships in which she consistently avoided support of an emotional nature.

It is noteworthy that as early as 1967, Beck argued in his seminal text on depression for the existence of latent cognitive schemata which become activated by the occurrence of specific events whose meaning are associated with those schemata. When applied to the present case, one might hypothesize that N.K.'s depression was strongly influenced by an affectively loaded cognitive schema originating from recurrent experiences of loss and emotional rejection. It is possible that this cognitive schema had been exacerbated at the time of childbirth and actively shaped the affective meaning of competent motherhood for this patient. Thus, it became critical for N.K. to provide a consistency in parenting which she had been deprived of throughout her childhood, while at the same time attempting to maintain her notion of competence by continuing to reject the support of others, especially her mother.

In addition to issues involving loss and emotional rejection, other developmental problems in a woman's childhood relationship with her own mother may lead to the formation of lasting cognitive schemata which become exacerbated during the transition to parenthood. For instance, the meaning of competent motherhood for a woman who as a child was abused by her mother often involves themes of whether she may abuse her own infant. Concerns about harming the infant may be experienced directly in automatic thoughts, less directly as excessive reactions to problems in affective attachment to the infant, or even more indirectly as persistent anxiety about the vulnerability of the infant and consequent hypervigilance.

In summary, when it appears that underlying cognitive schemata have been triggered by childbirth and have exerted an influence on postpartum depression, the therapist should assess the idiosyncratic manner in which the patient appraises her parenting experiences, and should evaluate whether there is an association between the patient's negative parenting appraisals and her basic constructs of self. When following this approach, therapy becomes less structured, less directive, and more protracted than in treatment targeted at the level of cognitive content. There is a greater focus on early developmental issues around parenting and the affective meaning that motherhood has for the patient. Returning to the treatment of N.K.,

> Therapy lasted for eleven months of weekly sessions. Treatment focused increasingly on helping N.K. to resolve her early deprivation experiences in a manner that allowed her to distinguish between the affective meaning she attached to parenting, the actual needs of her child, and her own legitimate needs as a parent for support. The patient gradually was able to allow her mother and husband to assist in childrearing more routinely and to experience less anxiety about the vulnerability of her baby. N.K. was able to reappraise her dysfunctional beliefs about herself so that accepting emotional support from others no longer represented a threat to her sense of competence.

## Recurrent Depressions

Differences in intervening at the levels of automatic thoughts and underlying schemata have been discussed. A third group of postpartum depressed patients are those who have experienced chronic or recurrent depressions in the past. In these cases the clinician's approach must broaden further. Prepartum affect, life event stressors, social supports, infant health and temperament, as well as cognitive content and schemata regarding motherhood, must all be assessed. In addition, the clinician should attempt to determine what factors contributed to prior depressions, whether they have been resolved, or whether they have reasserted their depressogenic influence at the time of childbirth. For instance, persistent problems in cognitive processing, such as self-blaming appraisals (Beck *et al.*, 1979) and negative internal attributions (Abramson *et al.*, 1978), are characteristic of the chronic depressive. During the perinatal period, the chronic depressive's self-blaming and negative internal attributional styles can be activated, contributing to perceptions of parenting inefficacy independent of actual performance. Moreover, memories unrelated to parenting *per se*, but involving themes of personal failure in other contexts, may be stimulated and lead to a further decline in postpartum affect. Additional problems with self-esteem and assertiveness, which are characteristic of these patients (Becker, 1979), may reduce their capacity to establish nurturant relationships from which they can draw support during stressful periods of parenthood. In these cases a treatment model which focuses only on parenting cognitions may be insufficient. Factors specific to the postpartum period must be incorporated into a broader treatment plan which utilizes interventions aimed at restructuring dysfunctional cognitive processes that have been developed by cognitive therapists for the chronic depressive (see Beck *et al.*, 1979).

A related problem involves pregnant patients who have experienced previous postpartum depression. These patients often are overcome by anxiety about how they will cope with another child and by fears that they will experience depression again. They may become hypervigilant to signs of dysphoria following childbirth and may interpret normal everyday postpartum mood fluctuations as evidence that they are beginning to experience another postpartum depression. It is not uncommon for their anxiety to reach a level where parenting performance actually is impaired. Moreover, these patients may appraise their previous postpartum depression as a failure and as evidence that they are poor mothers.

In such cases, the clinician should direct his/her efforts to helping the patient reframe her expectations and reduce her anxiety about her current perinatal experience. For instance, education about the normative aspects of postpartum mood fluctuations, and the difference between dysphoria and severe depression, often helps to reduce catastrophic appraisals of negative affect. Similarly, self-deprecating interpretations of a previous postpartum depression can sometimes be modified by encouraging the patient to reframe the episode as an important learning experience from which knowledge about how to prevent future depression can be gained.

## Cognitive Strategies for the Prevention
## of Postpartum Depression

Given that postpartum depression occurs within a relatively pre-
dictable time frame following childbirth, it might be possible to implement short-term prepartum interventions to reduce its prevalence (e.g.,
see Halonen & Passman, 1985). One strategy is to provide early intervention to patients identified at increased risk for postpartum depression based on the detection of risk factors (e.g., pregnancy depression,
poor spousal support, major life event stressors). The viability of this
approach depends on the clinician's ability to educate referral sources to
identify high-risk cases in the pregnant population. Since our own capacity to identify such cases based on research is still at a preliminary
stage, one can expect that even when referral relationships have been
developed, potential cases of postpartum depression will be missed. In
general, high-risk cases come to the attention of referral sources because
they already are experiencing significant problems during pregnancy,
such as depression, marital conflict, or ambivalence about becoming a
mother.

Pregnant patients who are identified at high risk can be assisted in
much the same manner as discussed in the therapy section of this chapter. Preventative strategies are determined by whether problems are
identified in cognitive content, motherhood-specific schemata, or are of
a recurrent depressive nature. Accordingly, prevention may focus on
education regarding parenting expectations, on historical explorations
of developmental issues around childrearing and their impact on parenting self-schemata, or on more standard therapy techniques to alter stable depressogenic cognitive processes, respectively. A major advantage
to offering interventions to high-risk cases prior to childbirth is that the
pregnant woman may have greater resources to apply to therapeutic
change. She is not yet burdened and preoccupied with the demands of
the newborn, or with the broader transitions that will occur in the family
unit after childbirth. In addition, having established a therapeutic relationship prepartum, the patient is less likely to hesitate in enlisting the
support of the clinician should postpartum difficulties develop.

As many women are unprepared for the multifaceted transitions
involved in becoming mothers, or in incorporating an additional child
into the family unit, a second prevention strategy is to offer prepartum
group education programs. These are aimed at providing information
about normative problems in postpartum adjustment and at shaping
expectations about obstetrical matters, maternal attachment, and parenting performance. The primary goal here is to encourage the develop-

ment of more flexible and realistic expectations prior to childbirth, so that patients are less likely to appraise their ability as parents on the basis of the commonly held, rigid ideals previously described. As the focus is on provision of education, and the active challenging of dysfunctional cognitions about parenting, the efficacy of such interventions depends on preselecting participants who are likely to experience problems primarily at the level of cognitive content. As noted previously, active educational interventions may not be effective when problems are at a schematic level involving developmental issues around motherhood. Moreover, chronic depressives require more intensive cognitive therapy approaches to address stable dysfunctional processes. History of good psychological adjustment and of a positive childhood relationship with the mother, as well as the absence of problems with recurrent depression, should be used as inclusion criteria for prepartum group education programs. In addition, cases involving prepartum high-risk factors may require more individually tailored attention than can be offered in a group education program.

The following is a summary of the interventions the author has found useful in running such groups in a local community hospital. Prepartum education ideally should include both prospective parents and should begin with a concerted attempt to debunk dysfunctional beliefs that parenthood is a stress-free, altogether joyful experience. While acknowledging positive aspects of parenting, it is important to emphasize the multifaceted levels of change that occur at the time of childbirth. Within this context, it is useful to reframe the transition to parenthood as a *crisis* requiring the development of attitudes and coping mechanisms which foster adaptation. For instance, participants should be encouraged to anticipate problems and disappointments with their pregnancies and deliveries. Rigid expectations that emotional bonding to the infant should follow a specific course which does not allow for ambivalent and negative affect need to be challenged. Myths that parenting expertise should come naturally have to be reappraised. Potential problems in these areas need to be decatastrophized and construed as part of normative experience, rather than as reflections of parenting inefficacy or personal failure.

Coping strategies should facilitate the development of a flexible outlook which recognizes the need for ongoing adaptation to respond to the baby's changing needs as maturation unfolds. It often is useful to emphasize that women may be increasing their risk for postpartum depression if they deprive themselves too much of personal reinforcement (e.g., Atkinson & Rickel, 1984) in order to conform to cultural stereotypes of selfless motherhood. Couples should be encouraged to consider how they intend to provide mutual support following child-birth. In addition, it is important to prepare couples for likely changes in their relationship. For instance, primiparous mothers often become en-amored and preoccupied with their infants during the early postpartum months and may be less invested in their relationships with their part-ners (Grossman *et al.*, 1980). As well, factors such as postdelivery physi-cal symptoms and the demands of the newborn can exhaust the new mother and reduce her interest in sexual relations. Marital conflicts may ensue if such changes are appraised as problems in the relationship, as opposed to normative experiences in adapting to parenting. Advance preparation may moderate against such appraisals and help to prevent the occurrence of postpartum depression as a result of loss of spousal support.

It should be emphasized that prepartum group education should be structured to allow for sufficient dialogue from participants so that the therapist can be sensitive to idiosyncratic expectations about parenting and can assess if adequate shifts occur in cognitive appraisal as a func-tion of interventions. An overly structured, didactic approach runs the risk of sensitizing participants to potential concerns without providing adequate opportunities for cognitive shifts and enhanced adaptation. Moreover, as in the case of N.K. described above, underlying dysfunc-tional schemata about motherhood only may become apparent when cognitive content about parenting is challenged. The clinician must be prepared to deal with the surfacing of such complicated cases in educa-tion groups, even when preselection criteria have been carefully ap-plied. Nonetheless, the detection of such cases may allow for early iden-tification of those in need of more intensive prepartum assistance.

## Summary

Over the last 15 years, there has been a growing interest in the phenomenon of postpartum depression. The clinical significance of postpartum depression is underscored by reports that it occurs in 10% to 20% of women, may persist throughout the first year after childbirth, and impacts on all members of the family unit. To date, research has focused on identifying vulnerability factors. Prepartum depression, poor spousal support, life event stressors, and infant health and tem-perament characteristics all appear to increase risk. How these variables interact to influence depression in individual cases is only beginning to be considered. There is some evidence that cognitive factors, such as self-appraisals of parenting competence, may increase vulnerability to postpartum depression and mediate the impact of other risk factors.

The phenomenology of postpartum depression is characterized by a preoccupation with the vulnerability of the infant, poor parenting self-efficacy, and broader appraisals that one is an inadequate mother. These perceptions may be affected by irrational expectations about obstetrical matters, maternal attachment, or parenting performance. In some cases, developmental issues involving the mother's own parenting become exacerbated at the time of childbirth, actively shaping the woman's identity as a mother and adding a level of idiosyncratic complexity to the meaning she attaches to parenting.

In this chapter, a cognitive model was outlined with which to conceptualize the phenomenology of postpartum depression. This model was influenced by the seminal work of Beck, Bandura, and Ellis, and by recent constructivist-based developments in cognitive therapy proposed by authors such as Guidano, Liotti, and Safran. Emphasis was placed on detailed assessment of the idiosyncratic nature of cognitive processes, identification of affectively loaded cognitions, exploration of developmental experiences, use of therapy process and the therapy relationship, and the distinctions between cognitive content and cognitive schemata. Based on this conceptual framework, guidelines for interventions with the postpartum depressed were outlined.

Many aspects of the present treatment model are speculative and require empirical validation. For instance, research is needed to determine whether problems in cognitive content and cognitive schemata can be reliably distinguished early in the clinical assessment of postpartum depressed patients. This is necessary for appropriate interventions to be applied based on an initial assessment of the level of cognitive dysfunction, rather than on a post hoc, trial-and-error basis. Moreover, well-controlled studies should be conducted to establish the optimal timing for specific interventions. While prevention may be the ideal goal, it remains to be demonstrated that prepartum cognitive interventions actually reduce the prevalence or severity of postpartum depression. In addition to such research endeavors, it is hoped that the present chapter will stimulate clinicians to consider applying their skills to the treatment of postpartum depression.

## REFERENCES

Abramson, L. Y., Seligman, M. E. P., & Teasdale, J. P. (1978). Learned helplessness in humans: Critique and reformulation. *Journal of Abnormal Psychology, 87,* 49-74.

Atkinson, A. K., & Rickel, A. U. (1984). Postpartum depression in primiparous parents. *Journal of Abnormal Psychology, 93,* 115-119.

Bandura, A. (1977). Self-efficacy: Toward a unifying theory of behavioral change. *Psychological Review, 84,* 191-215.

Bandura, A. (1982). Self-efficacy in human agency. *American Psychologist, 37*, 122-147.

Beck, A. T. (1967). *Depression: Causes and treatment*. Philadelphia: University of Pennsylvania Press.

Beck, A. T., Rush, A. J., Shaw, B. F., & Emery, G. (1979). *Cognitive therapy of depression*. New York: Guilford.

Becker, J. (1979). Vulnerable self-esteem as a predisposing factor in depressive disorders. In R. A. Depue (Ed.), *The psychobiology of the depressive disorders: Implications for the effects of stress* (pp. 317-334). New York: Academic Press.

Benedek, T. (1970). Motherhood and nurturing. In E. J. Anthony & T. Benedek (Eds.), *Parenthood: Its psychology and psychopathology* (pp. 153-165). Boston: Little, Brown.

Blumberg, N. L. (1980). Effects of neonatal risk, maternal attitude and cognitive style on early postpartum adjustment. *Journal of Abnormal Psychology, 89*, 139-150.

Bridge, L. R., Little, B. C., Hayworth, J., Dewhurst, S. J., & Priest, R. G. (1985). Psychometric ante-natal predictors of post-natal depresesed mood. *Journal of Psychosomatic Research, 29*, 325-331.

Cogill, S. R., Caplan, H. L., Alexandra, H., Robson, K. M., & Kumar, R. (1986). Impact of maternal postnatal depression on cognitive development of young children. *British Medical Journal, 292*, 1165-1167.

Cutrona, C. E. (1983). Causal attributions and perinatal depression. *Journal of Abnormal Psychology, 92*, 161-172.

Cutrona, C. E., & Troutman, B. R. (1986). Social support, infant temperament, and parenting self-efficacy: A mediational model of postpartum depression. *Child Development, 57*, 1507-1518.

Dalton, K. (1980). *Depression after childbirth*. New York: Oxford University Press.

Dix, C. (1985). *The new mother syndrome*. New York: Simon & Schuster.

Ellis, A. (1962). *Reason and emotion in psychotherapy*. New York: Lyle-Stuart.

Ellis, A. (1980). Rational-emotive therapy and cognitive-behavior therapy: Similarities and differences. *Cognitive Therapy and Research, 4*, 325-340.

Gelder, M. (1978). Hormones and postpartum depression. In M. Sandler (Ed.), *Mental illness in pregnancy and the puerperium* (pp. 80-90). Oxford: Oxford University Press.

Grossman, F. K., Eichler, L. S., & Winickoff, S. A. (1980). *Pregnancy, birth, and parenthood*. San Francisco: Jossey-Bass.

Guidano, V. F., & Liotti, G. (1983). *Cognitive processes and the emotional disorders*. New York: Guilford.

Guidano, V. F., & Liotti, G. (1988). A constructivistic foundation for cognitive therapy. In M. J. Mahoney & A. Freeman (Eds.), *Cognition and psychotherapy* (pp. 101-142). New York: Plenum.

Halonen, J. S., & Passman, R. H. (1985). Relaxation training and expectation in the treatment of postpartum distress. *Journal of Consulting and Clinical Psychology, 53*, 839-845.

Handley, S. L., Dunn, T. L., Waldron, G., & Baker, J. M. (1980). Tryptophan, cortisol and puerperal mood. *British Journal of Psychiatry, 136*, 498-508.

Heitler, S. K. (1976). *Postpartum depression: A multidimensional study*. Unpublished doctoral dissertation, New York University.

Hopkins, J., Marcus, M., & Campbell, S. B. (1984). Postpartum depression: A critical review. *Psychological Bulletin, 95*, 498-515.

Keating, G. W., & Manning, T. (1974). Infant temperament and sex of the infant: Effects on maternal behavior. In P. M. Shereshefsky & L. J. Yarrow (Eds.), *Psychological aspects of a first pregnancy and early postnatal adaptation* (pp. 225-236). New York: Raven Press.

Kendell, R. E. (1985). Emotional and physical factors in the genesis of puerperal mental disorders. *Journal of Psychosomatic Research, 29*, 3-11.

Kumar, R., & Robson, K. M. (1984). A prospective study of emotional disorders in childbearing women. *British Journal of Psychiatry, 144,* 35-47.

Leifer, M. (1977). Psychological changes accompanying pregnancy and motherhood. *Genetic Psychology Monographs, 95,* 55-96.

Liotti, G. (1987). The resistance to change of cognitive structures: A counterproposal to psychoanalytic metapsychology. *Journal of Cognitive Psychotherapy: An International Quarterly, 1,* 87-102.

Martin, M. (1977). A maternity hospital study of psychiatric illness associated with childbirth. *Irish Journal of Medical Science, 146,* 239-244.

O'Hara, M. W. (1986). Social support, life events, and depression during pregnancy and the puerperium. *Archives of General Psychiatry, 43,* 569-573.

O'Hara, M. W., Rehm, L. P., & Campbell, S. B. (1982). Predicting depressive symptomatology: Cognitive-behavioral models and postpartum depression. *Journal of Abnormal Psychology, 91,* 457-461.

O'Hara, M. W., Rehm, L. P., & Campbell, S. B. (1983). Postpartum depression: A role for social network and life stress variables. *Journal of Nervous and Mental Disease, 171,* 336-341.

Olioff, M., & Aboud, F. E. (in press). Predicting postpartum dysphoria in primiparous mothers: Roles of perceived parenting self-efficacy and self-esteem. *Journal of Cognitive Psychotherapy: An International Quarterly.*

Paykel, E. S., Emms, E. M., Fletcher, J., & Rassaby, E. S. (1980). Life events and social support in puerperal depression. *British Journal of Psychiatry, 136,* 339-346.

Pitt, B. (1968). Atypical depression following childbirth. *British Journal of Psychiatry, 114,* 1325-1335.

Rehm, L. P. (1977). A self-control model of depression. *Behavior Therapy, 8,* 787-804.

Safran, J. D., & Greenberg, L. S. (1986). Hot cognition and psychotherapy process: An information processing/ecological approach. In P. C. Kendall (Ed.), *Advances in cognitive-behavioral research and therapy* (Vol. 5, pp. 143-177). New York: Academic Press.

Safran, J. D., Vallis, T. M., Segal, Z. V., & Shaw, B. F. (1986). Assessment of core cognitive processes in cognitive therapy. *Cognitive Therapy and Research, 10,* 509-526.

Uddenberg, N., & Englesson, I. (1978). Prognosis of postpartum mental disturbance—a prospective study of primiparous women and their four-and-a-half-year-old children. *Acta Psychiatrica Scandinavica, 1958,* 201-212.

Wrate, R. M., Rooney, A. C., Thomas, P. F., & Cox, J. L. (1985). Postnatal depression and child development. A three-year follow-up study. *British Journal of Psychiatry, 146,* 622-627.

Youngs, D. D., & Lucas, M. J. (1980). Postpartum depression: Hormonal versus alternative perspectives. In D. D. Youngs & A. A. Ehrhardt (Eds.), *Psychosomatic obstetrics and gynecology* (pp. 29-38). New York: Appleton-Century-Crofts.

# 7

# The Application of Cognitive Therapy to the Bereaved

STEPHEN FLEMING AND PAUL J. ROBINSON

In the present chapter the application of cognitive-behavior therapy to the treatment of those who have experienced the death of a loved one is outlined. A cognitive-behavioral approach is of particular value in the treatment of the bereaved because of the focus on *personal meaning*—in this case, the personal meaning of the loss to the bereaved. Depending upon individual circumstances, this focus on personal meaning may take one or more forms. First, it may involve exploration of the bereaved's appraisal of the past, present, and hoped-for future relationship with the deceased. Second, it may entail the exploration of the bereaved's expectations with regard to his/her understanding of the grief process. Finally, focus on personal meaning may involve exploration of the meaning of the loss and its impact on the survivor's self-concept. Each of these foci receive more or less attention in therapy, depending upon the nature of the grief reaction and the therapist's conceptualization of the key therapeutic issues that warrant consideration.

In this chapter, a model of grief that provides an overview of the general response patterns to the death of a loved one will be presented. This model can be used to assist in the assessment and conceptualization of the nature of the grief reaction. Following the introduction of the model, specific cognitive-behavioral intervention strategies adapted for the bereaved will be discussed.

STEPHEN FLEMING • Department of Psychology, Atkinson College, York University, North York, Ontario M3J 2R7, Canada.     PAUL J. ROBINSON • Department of Psychology, North York General Hospital, Willowdale, Ontario M2K 1E1, Canada.

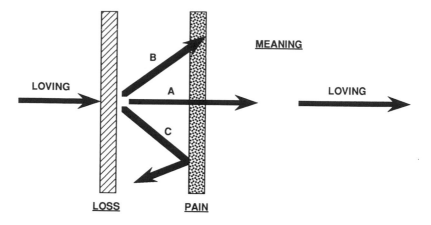

FIGURE 1. A model of the grief process: A, typical grief process; B, chronic grief process; C, delayed grief process.

## A MODEL OF GRIEF

### Description of the Model

We have developed a model of the grief process that is also a useful guide to intervention (Figure 1). Grief has been described as the transition of losing what we have to having what we have lost. That is, the experience of grief entails movement from resentment (losing what we have) to gratefulness (having what we have lost). The task of grieving, then, is to re-appraise the meaning of lost relationships.

In Figure 1, the term *pain* represents the host of complex physical, affective, cognitive, and behavioral responses to death (i.e., grief). It is important to note that grief is an expected, typical response to death and not necessarily a pathological reaction that requires professional intervention. It is the price we pay for loving. Typical, or uncomplicated grief, is characterized in Figure 1 by A. The survivor, in exploring such painful feelings as guilt, anger, sadness, anxiety, loneliness, and helplessness (i.e., processing his/her loss at a cognitive-affective level), eventually completes the tasks of mourning (Worden, 1982). The tasks or demands of grief, according to Worden (1982), involve accepting the reality of the loss, experiencing the pain of grief, adjusting to an environment in which the deceased is missing, and eventually, withdrawing emotional energy and reinvesting it in another relationship.

An appreciation by the bereaved of the legacy of the deceased is an important aspect of grief work and grief resolution. This legacy is painfully realized as the survivor grapples with such questions as, "What lessons in living has the deceased taught me?" "What lessons in loving have I learned?" "What has knowing and loving the deceased meant to me?" and "How am I different as a result of this intimate relationship?" The reappraisal of one's relationship with the deceased, and the consequent movement from resentment to gratefulness, is a highly emotionally charged process associated with the acknowledgment of the extent of one's loss.

The grief responses depicted in B and C in Figure 1 represent alternative styles of adjustment to loss. A chronic grief response (B) occurs when the survivor continuously exhibits intense reactions over an extended period of time (Parkes, 1986; Rando, 1984; Worden, 1982). These symptoms are more appropriate during the early phases of grief, but since there is an inability to relinquish emotional attachment to the deceased, the survivor is stuck. The therapeutic goal in this instance is to assist the bereaved in exploring and resolving the factors that are impeding the processing and integration of this loss experience (i.e., assist the bereaved to "say good-bye" to his/her pain). Factors such as fear of the future, guilt, dependency, or secondary gain, may impede this process.

The grief response depicted by C in Figure 1 applies when the survivor is aware of the loss, but for a variety of reasons inhibits, suppresses, or postpones the grief. Some reasons for this may include fear, lack of social support, multiple life stressors, the nature of the relationship with the deceased, or the personal meaning of the loss. With the inhibition or postponement of grief, the therapeutic goal is to assist the bereaved in acknowledging the affective dimensions of the loss (i.e., "say hello" to the pain). More specifically, the therapist helps the bereaved to identify factors preventing the full experience of the pain of the loss. Following this, the personal meaning of the death is explored, using a number of intervention strategies (see below).

It is important to stress that there is great variability in the adjustment to loss. In fact, as Zisook and Shuchter (1986) have noted, ". . . there is no prescription for how to grieve properly for a lost spouse, and no research-validated guideposts for what is normal versus deviant mourning. . . . We are just beginning to realize the full range of what may be considered 'normal' grieving" (p. 288). Wortman and Silver (1989), in critically evaluating many of the common assumptions underlying the grief process, have challenged and rejected the widely held beliefs that distress inevitably follows loss, that failure to experience distress is pathological, and that individuals recover from the death of a loved one within a limited period of time.

## Advantages of the Model

There are a number of characteristics of this model which make it particularly useful for understanding the nature and dynamics of the grief process. First, the necessity of assessing preloss personality, and the host of mediating variables that may affect the bereaved's response to the loss, is recognized. Assessment of the bereaved must include consideration of such factors as: the number, type, and quality of secondary losses; whether the death was sudden or expected; concurrent stressors; the characteristic style of handling stress; the bereaved's social, cultural, ethnic, and religious background; and the physical health of the bereaved (for a more detailed discussion of the myriad of factors influencing adjustment to loss, see Parkes, 1986; Rando, 1984).

Consideration of these mediating variables often results in a greater understanding of the struggle of the survivor, and less of an emphasis on pathology. To illustrate this point, consider the following case:

> C.S., a 48-year-old father of two adolescent children, was seen for a psychological assessment 18 months after the sudden death of his wife in a motor vehicle accident. Married 19 years, C.S. and his wife had been travelling in two separate vehicles along a rural road when his wife's vehicle collided with a hay wagon, killing her instantly. From the available, previously compiled psychological profiles, C.S. was diagnosed as having a complicated bereavement reaction on the basis of the length of time since the accident, his inability to talk about his wife without weeping, and his tendency to avoid talk of his wife within the family unit.

However, this diagnosis of complicated bereavement is questionable when one considers the following. First, using time as a measure of grief resolution is unreliable (Hoagland, 1984; Wortman & Silver, 1989). Second, C.S.'s characteristic style of dealing with emotionally volatile material was to be consistently uncomfortable, and to therefore avoid. Third, the constant exposure to lawyers, psychiatrists, and psychologists stemming from the litigation following the accident complicated C.S.'s emotional reaction. The reliving of the accident inherent in this process prevented C.S. from processing and integrating the loss (i.e., examining the legacy and the meaning of the relationship with his wife). Finally, the pressing demands of his professional life as an engineer, as well as the stresses of single parenthood, left little time for grieving. Collectively, these facts suggest that a diagnosis of C.S.'s grief is less important than understanding the factors mediating his grief. In Figure 1, then, the response styles represented by *B* and *C* can only be assessed, conceptualized, and treated after a thorough evaluation of the survivor's preloss personality, life history, and current life situation.

Another advantage of this model is a broadening of our understanding of what constitutes grief resolution. Whether using such terms as "reorganization" (Bowlby, 1980), "reintegration" (Raphael, 1983), or "withdrawing and reinvesting emotional energy" (Worden, 1982), there is a consensus that grief has a point of resolution with both cognitive (finding a rationale for the loss, understanding what has happened, making sense of the death) and affective components. With respect to the cognitive component of grief resolution, it is our opinion that survivors seldom, if ever, are able to make sense of a loss or find meaning in a death (this is particularly true when a child has died). You do not find meaning in *death*, you find meaning in the *life* that was lived. Central to the struggle to find meaning in the life that was lived is the notion of the deceased's legacy. The legacy is the appreciation of how knowing and loving the deceased has irrevocably changed the survivor, thus realizing the transition from losing what one has to having what one has lost. In this conceptualization, then, the cognitive focus in grief intervention is not in making sense of the death but, rather, finding meaning in the life that was lived, through appreciating the deceased's legacy. It must be stressed that the personal meaning of the loss can only be realized as a result of processing the affect associated with the death.

Finally, with respect to the resolution of grief, the therapist needs to gently explore the survivor's expectations of when the "end" will occur. There is mounting evidence that the period of active grieving is actually much longer than previously thought (Lehman, Wortman, & Williams, 1987).

In this model, it is recognized that dealing with the pain of loss and appreciating the legacy of the deceased frequently results in personality change and the restructuring of one's sense of self. The survivor's subsequent experiences in loving relationships will also differ from those relationships prior to the death. However, this personality restructuring need not occur with every loss experience. When the death involves a central figure in one's life, and when the death is seen as preventable (Bugen, 1979), the cognitive/affective upheaval is extensive, and this increases the likelihood of complications developing in the grieving process.

## The Importance of Affect in Grief

Since the alternative or atypical styles of dealing with one's grief involve either feeling overwhelmed by the affect (i.e., continually processing and reprocessing the affect) or avoiding it, affect is a primary focus when working with the bereaved. Recent discussions in the cognitive therapy literature by Greenberg and Safran (1987), Guidano and Liotti (1983), and Mahoney (1988) allow one to conceptualize the painful affect of grief as an ally when working with the bereaved. The emotional aspect of grief reflects a primitive and powerful form of knowing that should be explored, experienced, and expressed fully. As a result, the survivor recognizes feelings that may not have been experienced, or fully experienced, at the time of the loss because of their aversive properties.

As Averill (1968) and Bowlby (1980) have argued, the grief process is an adaptive, expected reaction to the loss of an important attachment figure. The emotional component of this reaction, as well as the other physical, behavioral, social, and cognitive manifestations of the grief process, are understandable and should be viewed as reflecting this adaptive process. The cognitive-behavior therapist who is working with the bereaved, therefore, will find that in contrast to the more structured, time-limited forms of cognitive therapy, a more flexible therapeutic approach is required.

## Cognitive-Behavioral Interventions

Prior to discussing specific cognitive-behavioral intervention strategies, an outline of our general approach to therapy with the bereaved will be presented. In most cases, the initial encounter with the bereaved person involves a review of the circumstances surrounding the death. A systematic study by Pennebaker and O'Heeron (1984) has confirmed the common clinical experience that the bereaved person benefits greatly from talking with another person about the circumstances of the death of the loved one. From this review, the therapist often begins to understand the nature of the survivor's affective, cognitive, and behavioral reactions. Therapists working with the bereaved individual should be prepared to tolerate the survivor's painful affective expression, as he/she details the nature of the death. Based partly on this expression, the therapist may then evaluate whether the person is typical, chronic, or delayed in response style, as outlined in Figure 1 (see Bowlby, 1980; Parkes, 1986; Rando, 1984; Schneider, 1980; and Worden, 1982, for further detailed discussions of the differentiation of these various reactions).

Once the bereaved has been provided with ample time to tell the story of the death, and encouraged to begin to fully express related thoughts and feelings, intervention usually proceeds with the introduction of educative material by the therapist. This material is usually presented regardless of the nature of the grief response. In fact, the survivor's response to this information may provide the therapist with further understanding of the individual's beliefs about the life and death of the deceased, as well as expectations of the grief process itself. In presenting educational material, then, the therapist obtains some degree of access to the affective and cognitive features of the survivor's grief reaction, and this sets the occasion for a number of intervention strategies. These interventions may include further affective exploration, the institution of appropriate behavioral techniques, and/or the direct consideration of the cognitive component of the grief reaction.

The remainder of this chapter will be devoted to specific educational, behavioral, and cognitive strategies that can guide grief therapy. Although these components will be separately presented, their interdependent and overlapping nature in the context of exploring the survivor's emotional response to loss in cognitive therapy must be recognized.

## The Educational Component

Grief, at times, may be experienced as frightening, overwhelming, even "crazy-making." To facilitate the full exploration of one's affective ties to the deceased, the survivor needs, as far as the therapist can provide, realistic information regarding common feelings and behaviors associated with loss. Although educating the bereaved will not result in the elimination of their anguish, it can normalize many of their unpredictable and painful emotional responses, and thereby reduce feelings of anxiety and helplessness. Often, this educational component is undertaken relatively early in therapy, although it can occur at any point.

In addition to suggesting readily available books on grief and adjustment (e.g., Knapp, 1986; Rando, 1988; Temes, 1980), the therapist can help the survivor to anticipate difficult emotional periods, and develop adaptive responses for these times. For example, when one considers the numerous, personally meaningful dates throughout the year (birthdays, anniversary of the death, wedding anniversaries, religious holidays, civic holidays, and other significant occasions), the calendar year represents a psychological minefield for which the bereaved is often ill-prepared.

The education of the bereaved and normalization of their experiences also provides an opportunity for both the therapist and the patient to understand the meaning attributed to the grief process by the patient. For example, the symptoms of grief may have a meaning that is particularly threatening to the bereaved individual. If he/she holds a belief that emphasizes the importance of inhibiting emotional expression (e.g., for fear of being hurt, or losing control), the affect-laden grief process may be too anxiety provoking, and the individual may misinterpret their grief experiences as the occurrence of the much-feared outcome. Thus, some bereaved individuals may appear avoidant of their grief, as they are frozen somewhere between the fear of emotional display and the grief-related demands of emotional acceptance and expression. In therapy, if progress is to be realized, attention has to be paid to the role of this often long-held belief in the complication of the bereavement reaction. In this case, the role of a belief regarding emotional inhibition in the avoidance of the grief work may have to be actively considered with the patient. A number of standard cognitive interventions to facilitate adaptive reappraisal of this belief are available to the cognitive therapist (Beck, Rush, Shaw, & Emery, 1979). From the educational component, therefore, a focus upon personal meaning very often begins to evolve.

For many survivors, an educational focus is sufficient to facilitate the grief work and the integration of the loss experience. For many others, however, behavioral and cognitive-behavioral strategies have to be implemented. This is often the case for those whose reaction to the death appears unusually delayed or chronic.

## The Behavioral Component

The most common behavioral interventions used in the treatment of problematic grief responses are flooding and graduated exposure (e.g., Gauthier & Pye, 1979; Ramsey, 1977). For example, noting a similarity between phobias and avoidant grief reactions, Ramsey (1977) advocates the use of techniques such as flooding, repeated confrontation, prolonged exposure, and response prevention when the bereaved client attempts to escape or avoid the pain of grief. In Ramsey's terms, the avoidance behavior of the bereaved is similar to that of the phobic, in that the stimuli that trigger the grief process (which, in turn, might elicit the responses necessary for extinction) are avoided. Gauthier and Marshall (1977) also reported on the use of flooding in the treatment of delayed grief responses.

Although the work reported by Ramsey (1977) and Gauthier and Marshall (1977) is limited due to its sole reliance on case studies, the authors of both of these studies report that the procedures were effective. It is likely, however, that for many individuals, the use of such an intensive procedure as flooding may not be desirable (Gauthier & Pye, 1979). Several authors and researchers, therefore, have discussed the use of a more graduated, less intensive procedure in the exposure of the bereaved to the grief-eliciting stimuli (e.g., Gauthier & Pye, 1979; Hodgkinson, 1982; Lieberman, 1978; Mawson, Marks, Ramm, & Stern, 1981; Melges & DeMaso, 1980; Turco, 1981).

Most of the graduated exposure approaches to the treatment of complicated bereavement have utilized a guided mourning procedure (e.g., Hodgkinson, 1982; Lieberman, 1978; Mawson *et al.*, 1981). Following an initial assessment of the individual, this procedure generally involves the repeated stimulation of the affect associated with the deceased to the point at which the bereaved demonstrates relief of the disruptive symptomatology that initially led to treatment. In contrast to flooding, however, this strategy is most often carried out at a pace and intensity less threatening to the patient. Nevertheless, exposure to the threatening emotion remains the focus and is often directly encouraged by the therapist by the use of what are called *linking objects* (Volkan, 1972). These are objects associated with the deceased toward which the bereaved has attributed special meaning (e.g., photographs, jewelry, clothing, etc.). The therapist also may encourage the bereaved to confront his/her grief outside of the therapy by prescribing visits to the cemetery, to the deceased's place of birth, or to any other situation that may stimulate the necessary grief work. Hodgkinson (1982) also reported the use of the Gestalt empty chair technique, in which the bereaved is encouraged to act out dialogues with the deceased.

The use of graduated exposure in the treatment of a grief response is illustrated in the following case:

> One of the authors (S.F.) utilized an exposure intervention in the treatment of L.B., a 55-year-old widow who had nursed her 28-year-old son at home, as he was dying from cancer. Her son was a concert pianist, who had recorded much of his own music. Although she loved classical music, following his death she could not listen to audiotapes of her son's recitals, nor derive much enjoyment from listening to any other classical music. With L.B.'s assistance, the therapist developed a list of composers ranging from those most unlike her son's favorite composer (Schumann) to her son playing Schumann. Following relaxation training, the therapist and L.B. worked through the hierarchy. Woven into this approach of systematic desensitization was attention to, and exploration of, the affective dimension of L.B.'s loss. Moreover, prior to the initiation of systematic desensitization, some time was spent assessing L.B.'s grief-related responses, allowing her the opportunity to review both the circumstances of the death and the nature of her relationship with her son.

A second case example illustrates the effectiveness of graduated exposure:

The same therapist worked with N.Y., a 24-year-old woman whose 18-month-old son had died when she drove through a stop sign and was hit by an oncoming truck. N.Y. was seen in therapy approximately eight months following the death of her son. Her primary complaint at the time of the initial therapeutic contact was that she was afraid to stay home alone (she had no other children). Her regular schedule included working from 9 A.M. to 5 P.M., and then travelling to her mother's house after work, where she would fall asleep on the sofa. Her husband would pick her up at her mother's house after he finished his 3 P.M. to 11:30 P.M. shift. As a result of the unsettled nature of this pattern, the levels of marital tension and individual irritability were growing increasingly higher.

Following a full exploration of the affective response to her child's death, including self-blame, *in vivo* exposure was implemented. Once a baseline of the length of time that N.Y. could stay home alone after 5 P.M. was determined, both the therapist and N.Y.'s husband would share the responsibility of phoning her near the end of this baseline period of time. During the call, N.Y. was urged to wander from the phone to other parts of the house, and her time period for staying at home gradually increased. Within three weeks, she was staying at home alone until her husband returned from work. Gradually, a more natural pattern of functioning returned, and eventually she became pregnant, and delivered a healthy baby boy.

As both of these case examples indicate, the behavioral component of a cognitive-behavioral approach can be an important aspect of the treatment of the bereaved. However, cognitive-behavior therapists are not only interested in the application of such procedures for the purposes of behavior change alone. They also attend to changes in beliefs that may result from the use of these methods (DeRubeis & Beck, 1988). Specifically, the personal meaning of the loss is one of the major areas that will change as the bereaved works through the grief process. Thus, in addition to the application of behavioral strategies in fostering this work, a number of cognitive features and interventions can be implemented.

## The Cognitive Component

Prior to outlining the cognitive features of grief that may require direct intervention, an overview of the relevant literature on cognition and bereavement is warranted. This discussion will be followed by a consideration of the erroneous expectations commonly held by the bereaved, the paradoxes of grief, the role of rigid beliefs, and the importance of attending to levels of cognitive processes.

Although there are relatively few studies of cognitive therapy with the bereaved, several authors have offered pertinent theoretical discussions or clinical case studies (Abrahms, 1981; Bowlby, 1980; Hoagland, 1984; Woodfield & Viney, 1984-85). As well, numerous researchers have considered the nature of cognition in the adjustment to loss (e.g., Bornstein, Clayton, Halikas, Maurice, & Robins, 1973; Clayton, Herjanic, Murphy, & Woodruff, 1974; Gallagher, Dessonville, Breckenridge, Thompson, & Amaral, 1982; Lindemann, 1944; Parkes, 1965; Robinson & Fleming, 1989a, 1989b). Based on a selective review of systematic research focusing on the typical reaction of a person to the death of a spouse, and the manner in which this reaction differs from a depressive disorder, Robinson and Fleming (1989b) concluded that grief and depression rarely are similar in terms of extent of pathology in cognitive functioning.

Several researchers, including Abrahms (1981), Bornstein *et al.* (1973), Clayton *et al.* (1974), Gallagher *et al.* (1982), Horowitz *et al.* (1980), Lindemann (1944), Parkes (1965), and Robinson and Fleming (1989a), have highlighted the role of persistent, distorted, and negative perceptions of self, experience, and future, in the differentiation of major depression from a typical bereavement reaction. The Robinson and Fleming (1989a) study, however, is the only one that involved the use of instruments specifically designed to measure cognitive functioning. In this study, depressotypic cognitive patterns were compared in two groups of conjugally bereaved subjects (depressed and nondepressed), two groups of nonbereaved psychiatric inpatients (depressed and nondepressed), and a group of nonbereaved, nonpsychiatric (nondepressed) control subjects. The following three cognitive measures were administered: the Automatic Thoughts Questionnaire (ATQ; Hollon & Kendall, 1980), the Cognitive Errors Questionnaire (CEQ; Lefebvre, 1981), and the 100-item Dysfunctional Attitudes Scale (DAS; Weissman & Beck, 1978). In addition to completing these scales, as well as the Beck Depression Inventory (BDI; Beck, Ward, Medelson, Mock, & Erbaugh, 1961), all subjects initially participated in a structured interview (the Structured Clinical Interview for DSM-III; Spitzer & Williams, 1984) and were classified as to whether or not they met the criteria for depression.

The results of this study indicated that although the nondepressed bereaved showed levels of cognitive dysfunction similar to the nonbereaved, nonpsychiatric controls on the DAS and the CEQ, the nondepressed bereaved demonstrated more frequent negative automatic thoughts (as measured by the ATQ) than the controls. In turn, while the depressed bereaved manifested a greater frequency of negative automatic thoughts (on the ATQ) than did the nondepressed bereaved, they unexpectedly showed significantly lower frequencies than those obtained by the psychiatric depressed. This was unexpected, because both the depressed bereaved and the psychiatric depressed groups had met the interview criteria for major depressive disorder. Also unexpected was the finding that the two bereaved groups demonstrated similarly low cognitive dysfunction in terms of attitudes and errors (as measured by the DAS and the CEQ). Their level of cognitive dysfunction on these scales was no different than that displayed by the control subjects or the psychiatric nondepressed patients. All of these groups displayed significantly lower cognitive dysfunction on these measures than did the psychiatric depressed.

Collectively, these data indicate that although bereaved subjects (i.e., both those who met the criteria for depression, and those who did not) reported a greater frequency of negative automatic thoughts than did control subjects (as measured by the ATQ), these accessible thoughts were not anchored in corresponding cross-situational, depressive assumptions about the self, world, and future (as measured by the DAS and CEQ). The cognitive disruption in bereavement, therefore, may be superficial, situation-specific, and not necessarily anchored at an assumptive or global level, in contrast to what is seen with nonbereaved depressives.

These data also indicated that in spite of receiving the same diagnosis of major depression (via structured interview), the depressed bereaved did not display the high level of cognitive dysfunction displayed by the psychiatric depressed. Researchers in the area of cognition and depression (e.g., Hammen, Jacobs, Mayol, & Cochran, 1980; Krantz & Hammen, 1979) argue that when one identifies depression without dysfunctional cognitive bias, this affective disturbance is more benign than depression with cognitive bias. Thus, the depressed bereaved in our study appeared to be experiencing this less pathological affective experience. Clearly, a major depressive episode following bereavement is not equivalent, at least at a cognitive level, to a major depressive episode unassociated with bereavement.

In line with these inferences, it is our clinical experience that the choice of intervention strategy with the bereaved, at least in part, is a function of the ongoing assessment of the level and extent of cognitive disruption that has occurred. In particular, if the bereaved displays a style of grieving that is either chronic or delayed (see Figure 1), this raises the possibility that assumptive, self-related meaning structures are involved, and, therefore, these meaning structures may have to be targeted for intervention.

Bowlby (1980) has discussed the role of cognitive structures in chronic and delayed grief, as well as in healthy adaptation to the death of a loved one. In the case of a healthy outcome following bereavement, Bowlby argues that the bereaved likely possesses a representational model of attachment figures as available, responsive, and helpful, as well as a model of self as a lovable and valuable person. Moreover, the healthy bereaved is likely not afraid of affective expression. Thus, at the time of the death of the loved one, the bereaved grieves deeply, but will not hold (to any extent) a sense of self as rejected, nor will he/she manifest self-reproach. This observation is in line with Freud's (1917/ 1957) notion that negative self-regard is what differentiates depression from sadness or grief (i.e., it is absent in a typical grief process).

Bowlby (1980) argues that every situation in life is construed in terms of representational models of world and self. There may be certain situations, however, that one will find particularly difficult to process, such as when new information (the death of a loved one) clashes with established models (that include the existence and relationship with the loved one). In the face of such an experience, old representations gradually must be modified or replaced with new ones.

Based on a personal construct perspective, Hoagland (1984) and Woodfield and Viney (1984-85) concur with Bowlby that the death of a close other may invalidate much of the bereaved's construct system, and thus, large subsystems of constructs may require modification. Woodfield and Viney (1984-85) further argue that the bereaved vary in terms of the adaptability of their construct systems which, in turn, may affect the adjustment to the loss. Thus, if the bereaved have defined self and meaning in life in terms of the deceased and their relationship, the bereaved may become a "prisoner" of their construct system. Conversely, the bereaved whose prior beliefs about themselves and their relationships have encompassed a perspective broader than one based largely on the deceased, may adapt to the loss in a more satisfactory manner.

In light of the extent to which cognitive features appear to play a role in adjustment to loss, it follows that attention to the cognitive component in treatment is valuable. In addition to a consistent awareness and sensitivity on the part of the therapist to the likelihood that the bereaved may have to undertake a significant reorganization of his/her personal construct system (the survivor's awareness of which markedly increases his/her anxiety level; Kelly, 1955), a number of cognitive features of grief may warrant direct exploration and intervention. Such features include erroneous or dysfunctional expectations, paradoxical beliefs, rigid beliefs (shoulds, self-criticism, and guilt), and levels of cognitive disruption.

## Erroneous Expectations

Widely shared and erroneous expectations concerning the nature and dynamics of the grief response often increase the probability of complications developing. The therapist needs to assess for the presence of these misconceptions and be prepared to directly intervene. The most damaging misunderstandings tend to reflect a perception that grief is time limited (the phrase "time heals" portrays this belief). If the survivor, mirroring the expectations of well-meaning friends and society as a whole, expects that there is a point in time at which one "gets over" the death of a loved one (i.e., the feelings vanish), problems can develop when the feelings remain longer than the bereaved, or others, might expect.

Survivors often feel a puzzling, painful array of overwhelming emotional and physical responses, and frequently experience a loss of self-confidence during this tumultuous period. They may attribute the lack of synchrony between the internal reality of their grief and societal expectations of what they "should" be feeling at a particular point in time to their ineffective grieving style. At such times, there is a danger that grief will be suppressed, and feelings and behaviors more consistent with the expectations of others will be adopted. For example, others may think that it is time for a bereaved woman to begin dating again, and although she may not at all desire to participate in such an activity, she may attempt to ignore her genuine feelings, and seek out a date. This premature abandonment of one's true feelings often leads to damaging self-criticism and guilt (e.g., she reflects "How can I be on a date when my husband just died?").

In order to circumvent this potentially destructive situation, it is important to assist the bereaved in challenging such fallacies as "time heals." For instance, this expectation implies that the bereaved need not do anything, that simply the passage of time will lead to resolution. Grief, however, is anything by passive. The survivor needs to be gently made aware that it is not the time you have to use that dictates the course of grief, but rather how you use the time you have. In reality, one does not "get over" (i.e., forget) the death of a loved one, but, instead, one learns to "live with" the death of a loved one (i.e., to integrate the death and the life of the loved one into one's personal construct system). By discussing a more functional expectation of gradually increased periods of peacefulness and progressive release from the intense pain as the grief work proceeds, the therapist can facilitate the bereaved's reappraisal of such expectations.

### The Paradoxes of Grief

It is our clinical observation that the grief experience in some ways is contradictory or paradoxical. Thus, discussing these paradoxes with the bereaved can further provide them with a frame of reference for their experience and assist in the development of increasingly adaptive expectations. In turn, once these paradoxes are explored, the bereaved often will experience increased tolerance and acceptance of the "craziness" of grief.

It is not at all unusual for the bereaved to attribute their sometimes contradictory experiences in grief to a loss of control or, in their words, to "going crazy." The following paradoxes are examples of the type that characterize the experience of many survivors:

*"You will get worse before you get better."* In other words, it is necessary to experience the full affective response to the loss, and appreciate the legacy of the deceased, before the affective/cognitive upheaval of grief abates.

*"To regain your independence, allow yourself to be dependent."* Unrealistic expectations of independent functioning, without consideration for the weighty toll grief extracts, deprive the survivor of the solace friends bring. Allowing others to care for the bereaved (permitting a dependency), however temporary or therapeutic, may be threatening to many.

*"To 'let go' you have to be convinced the memory will stay."* Unable to recall the deceased's smile, voice, or clearly recollect a treasured memory, the survivor may catastrophize (e.g., "If I can't recall their voice at this moment, what will it be like a year from now I will have forgotten them completely!"). The resulting fear and panic over the prospect of forgetting can lead to a virtual obsession with the deceased. Memories are constantly processed, times together relentlessly recalled, as the survivor labors under the impossible expectation of readily recollecting "every waking moment" of their lives together. Assurance must be forthcoming from the therapist that just as one cannot recall every waking moment with those currently in our lives, one cannot recall every waking moment with our dead. Nevertheless, one does not "forget"; the memories are accessible.

*"You may not want to be with others, yet you don't want to be alone."* This paradox comes from C. S. Lewis (1961), who wrote, "I find it hard to take in what anyone says. Or perhaps, hard to want to take it in. It is so uninteresting. Yet I want the others to be about me. I dread the mo-

ments when the house is empty. If only they would talk to one another and not to me" (p. 7). Survivors often respond with relief when this puzzling, often contradictory, experience is validated by the therapist.

As noted above, the timely identification and discussion of these paradoxes may assist the bereaved in developing a more functional attribution of their experience. For example, as outlined by Abramson, Seligman, and Teasdale (1978) in their reformulation of the learned helplessness model of depression, rather than attributing their paradoxical experience to internal (personal), stable, and global factors (e.g., "I am crazy and will never recover"), the bereaved may reattribute their experience as external, unstable, and specific (e.g., "These are normal feelings in grief, and gradually I will feel less distressed and mixed up"). As some research has indicated, such a reattribution may leave an individual less vulnerable to depression (e.g., Golin, Sweeney, & Schaeffer, 1981; Peterson, Villanova, & Rapps, 1985). Beck *et al.* (1979) have also observed the usefulness of reattribution in the case of individuals who unrealistically attribute adverse occurrences to a personal deficiency.

## Rigid Beliefs

In addition to erroneous and paradoxical beliefs, another common cognitive feature of bereavement is the presence of rigid, dysfunctional beliefs expressed as "should" statements. Examples of such statements include: "I should be able to concentrate by now," "I should not still be crying," or "I should not be angry at my wife, she did not want to die." Consistent with rational-emotive techniques (e.g., Dryden & Ellis, 1986, 1988), assisting the bereaved in the elimination of such destructive beliefs and expectations may be accomplished through writing a prescription for the survivor (e.g., "Don't should yourself"). Alternatively, the therapist may encourage substitution for should statements (e.g., replacing "I should be able to concentrate for longer periods" with "I am currently unable to concentrate for lengthy periods"), or support the bereaved in challenging their own shoulds (e.g., "Who says I should? Where is it written that I should . . . ?").

Dryden and Ellis (1988) argue that absolutistic cognitions, such as should statements, often impede people in the pursuit of their basic goals and purposes. Indeed, such cognitions may lead to feelings of guilt, as people label themselves in a negative manner for not living up to these self-imposed expectations. For example, a widow may evidence self-criticism in the form of "I should have been a better wife to him, and since I wasn't, I am a rotten person" and experience a sense of guilt in relation to such a thought. Since it has been postulated that self-referent cognitions may indicate potential core or central cognitive dysfunction (Guidano & Liotti, 1983; Safran, Vallis, Segal, & Shaw, 1986), it is advised that the therapist pay close attention to such features when they occur in treatment. Whether the self-criticism and related guilt are anchored in dysfunctional, core cognitive structures is often only apparent as one attempts to intervene directly.

A number of cognitive interventions can be very useful in assisting the bereaved in the expression and resolution of self-criticism and guilt associated with the death of a loved one. Guilt may be objective (e.g., the bereaved actually may be guilty of involvement in the death, as determined by a court of law) or subjective, as was the case for N.Y., the woman whose 18-month-old child was killed in a motor vehicle accident (see above). In this latter instance, it is quite common for highly destructive labels to be applied by the bereaved to themselves (e.g., "I killed my child"). Eventually, the label itself is consistently applied to oneself (e.g., "I am a murderer"), with obvious condemning and depression-inducing consequences.

The first step in working with such extensive self-criticism is for both the therapist and the patient to examine the goals of intervention. It is unrealistic for either the therapist or the patient to anticipate that the final outcome will be a guilt-free reflection on the cause of the accident. Rather, the best one may hope for is manageable guilt, without complete self-condemnation. A general approach to this problem begins with affective exploration of the guilt, including the process of arriving at the label (e.g., "killer" or "murderer," in the case of N.Y.). A useful cognitive intervention is to examine the crucial ingredients that went into formulating the label (e.g., focus on such criteria as intent to do harm), and then have the bereaved explore the impact of this new information on the accuracy of the label. This process appeals to the logic that if one did not intend to do harm (intent is crucial to the use of the label "killer"), then there are other labels that might more accurately describe the situation, labels with less self-destructive and depressive potential. One might decide on applying such labels as "careless" or "unthinking," which are not only more accurate, but also less self-defeating. The most realistic goal in therapy is a reduction of the self-criticism and guilt to tolerable levels, not complete elimination of it.

## Levels of Cognitive Processes

If the above-mentioned approach to the occurrence of self-criticism yields little progress (i.e., the intervention has failed), attention to the levels of cognitive processes may assist in the formulation of an appropriate therapeutic direction. Specifically, self-related criticism may be resistant to change because it involves cognitions that are more central for an individual (Bugental & Bugental, 1984; Liotti, 1987; Mahoney, 1988; Safran et al., 1986). As noted by Safran et al. (1986), the occurrence of a failed intervention may indicate that the therapist unwittingly has challenged a core belief, provided of course that there is additional evidence to suggest that this belief is core. Bugental and Bugental (1984) also argue that the possibility of changing a core view of self elicits a threat to one's sense of identity and may be actively resisted. As has been argued in Chapter 3 (this volume), resistance to changing core beliefs may be self-protective (see also Liotti, 1987; Mahoney, 1988).

Cognitive interventions with the bereaved at times require a focus beyond cognitive content (e.g., the relabeling strategy described above) to a focus on the role of central, self-related cognitive structures. In addition to failed intervention as a possible marker of the operation of such structures, chronic or delayed grief may also indicate resistance to working through the grief process that is related to fundamental, self-related meaning structures. In light of the myriad mediating factors that can lead to alternative grieving styles (e.g., presence of secondary losses, social, religious background, etc.), however, it is important to assess for these prior to assuming that structural factors are the central problem.

It is relevant to acknowledge that therapeutic intervention at the level of cognitive structures (see Chapters 1 and 2, this volume, for a discussion of cognitive content, process, and structure) appears neither necessary nor appropriate for those bereaved who do not demonstrate complications at this level. As noted by Guidano and Liotti (1983), ". . . not every patient requires a 'deep' change in his or her cognitive organization. 'Superficial' or 'peripheral' changes in a reasonably adaptive paradigm are sometimes sufficient" (p. 160). It is our clinical experience that for many bereaved, especially those whose grief response is relatively uncomplicated, the expression and validation of their "crazy" thoughts is all that is required for significant anxiety reduction. Moreover, they tend to evidence progress in their grief when the behavioral and cognitive strategies already outlined are applied.

In contrast to those survivors who seem to manifest no core or deep structural difficulties, the issue of personal meaning should be explored in detail, if assessment indicates that the bereaved's automatic thoughts are anchored in maladaptive, core cognitive structures. The meaning of the loss vis-à-vis the self often becomes the central focus. In particular, in the case of delayed or chronic responses to loss, attention to such matters may be fundamental to assisting the bereaved in progressing with their grief work. To remain only at the level of thought content, and not attend to the levels of cognitive process and structure (particularly self-related), may lead to only limited therapeutic progress with these individuals. Even in the case of what appears to be a relatively uncomplicated bereavement, assessing the impact of the loss on the bereaved's self-perception is recommended (although, as noted above, intervention at this level is not always required).

Safran *et al.* (1986) have provided a number of guidelines for assessing the role of core cognitive processes in cognitive therapy. How this assessment may be undertaken, and the importance of focussing on self-related constructs in the evaluation of a bereavement reaction, is illustrated in the following case history provided by one of the authors (P.R.).

> S.A. was hospitalized due to the development of depressive symptomatology and suicidal ideation following the suicide of his wife. Many years earlier, he had been hospitalized due to depression, following a separation from another woman. During an early interview with S.A., he stated that he was responsible for his wife's death because he "should" have known that she was feeling this way and obtained help for her.

Such self-blame and accompanying guilt often is found for those who are struggling with their grief following the suicide of a loved one (Dunn & Morris-Vidners, 1988; Rando, 1984; Worden, 1982). It is helpful to explore the extent to which this often-found feature reflects profoundly negative and extensive self-perceptions. Thus, the automatic thought "I *should* have known . . . " may be conceptualized as a typical symptom of grief following the suicide of a close other, and explored no further. Alternatively, the therapist might conceptualize such an automatic thought as the focus of treatment and begin to dispute the "unrealistic" level of self-blame (e.g., "What is your evidence that you should have known?" "How would you have known that she would attempt to take her own life?"). In order to obtain sufficient information to allow the cognitive therapist to choose between several possible conceptualizations (e.g., the content versus structural level), we recommend against an early disputational approach (e.g., Dryden & Ellis, 1986; Ellis, 1981), and instead recommend detailed exploration of the meaning of the death vis-à-vis the self (the technique of vertical exploration; Safran *et al.*, 1986). Especially in the assessment phase, and early in therapy, one needs to continue to explore the survivor's thoughts and feelings fully, and not assist them in disputing their responses too early. The purpose of this approach is to assess the individual's self-evaluative activity in its totality.

> Thus, in the case of S.A., he was asked what it meant about *him* that he did not know his wife was going to kill herself. He replied that this meant that he was insensitive and unloving which, in turn, led him further to reveal

profound feelings of worthlessness and decreased self-esteem. He justi-
fied this judgment of self by pointing to his wife's suicide as rejection of
him, and indicated a fundamental view of himself as unlovable. His wife's
suicide had reactivated what appeared to be a tacit, central construct of self
as unlovable.

If one had quickly challenged this man at a content level (i.e., whether
he should have known that his wife was going to commit suicide), initial
understanding and subsequent intervention may have been less accurate and powerful. Understanding the nature of his self-related beliefs
alerted the therapist to the possibility that therapy may require a consideration of both the meaning of the loss, as well as the bereaved's
sense of self. The presence of chronic or delayed grief reactions, in
particular, may indicate this treatment possibility (see Chapter 1, this
volume, for a comparison of content-focused versus structure-focused
cognitive therapy).

## Summary and Conclusions

Cognitive-behavior therapy is of particular value in the treatment of
the bereaved because of the focus on *personal meaning*. Although there
are many features and strategies of cognitive-behavior therapy that do
not require modification when applied to problematic grief responses,
application to this population does demand increased flexibility on the
part of the therapist. In particular, therapists may spend more time
exploring the affective experience of the bereaved, as well as attending
to and working with the various facets and levels of the personal meaning of the loss.

Our review of the relevant cognitive-behavior techniques utilized in
therapy with the bereaved has been developed largely from clinical
work. As Wortman and Silver (1989) noted in their recent review of the
empirical research related to coping with loss, there is a need to evaluate
the validity of theoretical and clinical assumptions by the use of data-
based research. This observation certainly is pertinent to the application
of an established therapeutic approach to a novel population. As noted
by Dobson (1988), in his discussion of the future of cognitive-behavior
therapy, there is a continual need for research that documents the ap-
propriateness of expansions of therapeutic approaches.

With regard to the application of cognitive-behavior therapy to the
bereaved, it will be necessary to systematically consider under what
circumstances, and with what type of grief response, various cognitive-
behavioral approaches will be more or less helpful. This task is compli-

cated by two major factors. First, bereavement reactions and grief are only beginning to be understood by researchers (e.g., Wortman & Silver, 1989; Zisook & Shuchter, 1986). Second, cognitive-behavior therapy continues to undergo substantial development and diversification (Mahoney, 1988). Nonetheless, given these developments, it will be necessary to investigate which of these approaches is useful for which type of person, and under what circumstances.

Although many of the standard cognitive therapies and related strategies (e.g., Beck *et al.*, 1979) are directly applicable in the treatment of the bereaved, recent refinements and expansions in cognitive-behavior therapy may be of particular relevance and value. For example, therapeutic developments that encourage the expression and exploration of affect, and consider affect not as a problem but, rather, as a powerful knowing process and ally in therapy, seem valuable in the treatment of grief-related issues (e.g., Greenberg & Safran, 1987; Guidano & Liotti, 1983; Mahoney, 1988). This orientation may be especially relevant when the affective component of the grief process is delayed or chronic. In addition, when the grief reaction suggests the possibility that core-organizing schemata are challenged, approaches emphasizing increased attention to the differentiation of core versus peripheral cognitive structures seem particularly relevant (e.g., Guidano & Liotti, 1983; Safran *et al.*, 1986).

ACKNOWLEDGMENTS. The authors would like to thank Rheba Adolph for her contribution to the section "The Paradoxes of Grief."

# REFERENCES

Abrahms, J. (1981). Depression versus normal grief following the death of a significant other. In G. Emery, S. Hollon, & R. Bedrosian (Eds.), *New directions in cognitive therapy* (pp. 255-270). New York: Guilford.

Abramson, L., Seligman, M., & Teasdale, J. (1978). Learned helplessness in humans: Critique and reformulation. *Journal of Abnormal Psychology, 87*, 102-109.

Averill, J. (1968). Grief: Its nature and significance. *Psychological Bulletin, 70*, 721-748.

Beck, A., Ward, C., Mendelson, M., Mock, J., & Erbaugh, J. (1961). An inventory for measuring depression. *Archives of General Psychiatry, 4*, 561-571.

Beck, A. T., Rush, A. J., Shaw, B., & Emery, G. (1979). *Cognitive therapy of depression.* New York: Guilford.

Bornstein, P., Clayton, P., Halikas, J., Maurice, W., & Robins, E. (1973). The depression of widowhood after thirteen months. *British Journal of Psychiatry, 122*, 561-566.

Bowlby, J. (1980). *Attachment and loss* (Vol. 3). New York: Basic Books.

Bugen, L. (1979). Human grief: A model for prediction and intervention. In L. Bugen (Ed.), *Death and dying: Theory, research, and practice* (pp. 33-45). Dubuque, IA: W. C. Brown.

Bugental, J., & Bugental, E. (1984). A fate worse than death: The fear of changing. *Psychotherapy, 21*, 543-549.

Clayton, P., Herjanic, M., Murphy, G., & Woodruff, R. (1974). Mourning and depression: Their similarities and differences. *Canadian Psychiatric Association Journal, 19,* 309-312.

DeRubeis, R., & Beck, A. (1988). Cognitive therapy. In K. Dobson (Ed.), *Handbook of cognitive-behavioral therapies* (pp. 273-306). New York: Guilford.

Dobson, K. (1988). The present and future of the cognitive-behavioral therapies. In K. Dobson (Ed.), *Handbook of cognitive-behavioral therapies* (pp. 387-414). New York: Guilford.

Dryden, W., & Ellis, A. (1986). Rational-emotive therapy (RET). In W. Dryden & W. Golden (Eds.), *Cognitive-behavioral approaches to psychotherapy* (pp. 129-168). New York: Harper & Row.

Dryden, W., & Ellis, A. (1988). Rational-emotive therapy. In K. Dobson (Ed.), *Handbook of cognitive-behavioral therapies* (pp. 214-272). New York: Guilford.

Dunn, R., & Morrish-Vidners, D. (1988). The psychological and social experience of suicide survivors. *Omega: Journal of Death and Dying, 18,* 175-215.

Ellis, A. (1981). The rational-emotive approach to thanatology. In H. Sobel (Ed.), *Behavior therapy in terminal care: A humanistic approach* (pp. 151-176). Cambridge, MA: Ballinger.

Freud, S. (1957). Mourning and melancholia. In J. Strachey (Ed. and Trans.), *The standard edition of the complete psychological works of Sigmund Freud* (Vol. 14, pp. 243-258). London: Hogarth Press. (Original work published 1917).

Gallagher, D., Dessonville, C., Breckenridge, J., Thompson, L., & Amaral, P. (1982). Similarities and differences between normal grief and depression in older adults. *Essence, 5* 127-140.

Gauthier, J., & Marshall, W. (1977). Grief: A cognitive-behavioral analysis. *Cognitive Therapy and Research, 1,* 39-44.

Gauthier, J., & Pye, C. (1979). Graduated self-exposure in the management of grief. *Behavioral Analysis & Modification, 3,* 202-208.

Golin, S., Sweeney, P., & Schaeffer, D. (1981). The causality of causal attributions in depression: A cross-lagged panel correlation analysis. *Journal of Abnormal Psychology, 90,* 14-22.

Greenberg, L., & Safran, J. (1987). *Emotion in psychotherapy: Affect, cognition, and the process of change.* New York: Guilford.

Guidano, V., & Liotti, G. (1983). *Cognitive processes and emotional disorders.* New York: Guilford.

Hammen, C., Jacobs, M., Mayol, A., & Cochran, S. (1980). Dysfunctional cognitions and the effectiveness of skills and cognitive-behavioral assertion training. *Journal of Consulting and Clinical Psychology, 48,* 685-695.

Hoagland, A. (1984). Bereavement and personal constructs: Old theories and new concepts. In F. Epting & R. Neimeyer (Eds.), *Personal meanings of death* (pp. 89-107). New York: Hemisphere/McGraw-Hill.

Hodgkinson, P. (1982). Abnormal grief: The problem of therapy. *British Journal of Medical Psychology, 55,* 29-34.

Hollon, S., & Kendall, P. (1980). Cognitive self-statements in depression: Development of an automatic thoughts questionnaire. *Cognitive Therapy and Research, 4,* 383-395.

Kelly, G. (1955). *The psychology of personal constructs* (Vol. 1). New York: W. W. Norton.

Knapp, R. (1986). *Beyond endurance.* New York: Schocken.

Krantz, S., & Hammen, C. (1979). Assessment of cognitive bias in depression. *Journal of Abnormal Psychology, 88,* 611-619.

Lefebvre, M. (1981). Cognitive distortion and cognitive errors in depressed psychiatric and low back pain patients. *Journal of Consulting and Clinical Psychology, 49,* 517-525.

Lehman, D., Wortman, C., & Williams, A. (1987). Long-term effects of losing a spouse or child in a motor vehicle crash. *Journal of Personality and Social Psychology, 52,* 218-231.

Lewis, C. S. (1961). *A grief observed*. London: Faber & Faber.

Lieberman, S. (1978). Nineteen cases of morbid grief. *British Journal of Psychiatry, 132,* 159-163.

Lindemann, E. (1944). Symptomatology and management of grief. *American Journal of Psychiatry, 101,* 141-148.

Liotti, G. (1987). The resistance to change of cognitive structures: A counterproposal to psychoanalytic metapsychology. *Journal of Cognitive Psychotherapy: An International Quarterly, 1,* 87-104.

Mahoney, M. (1988). The cognitive sciences and psychotherapy: Patterns in a developing relationship. In K. Dobson (Ed.), *Handbook of cognitive-behavioral therapies* (pp. 357-386). New York: Guilford.

Mawson, D., Marks, I., Ramm, L., & Stern, R. (1981). Guided mourning for morbid grief: A controlled study. *British Journal of Psychiatry, 138,* 185-193.

Melges, F., & DeMaso, D. (1980). Grief-resolution therapy: Reliving, revising, and revisiting. *American Journal of Psychotherapy, 34,* 51-61.

Parkes, C. (1965). Bereavement and mental illness: Part 1—A clinical study of the grief of bereaved psychiatric patients. *British Journal of Medical Psychology, 38,* 1-12.

Parkes, C. M. (1986). *Bereavement: Studies of grief in adult life* (2nd ed.). New York: Penguin Books.

Pennebaker, J., & O'Heeron, R. (1984). Confiding in others and illness rate among spouses of suicide and accidental-death victims. *Journal of Abnormal Psychology, 93,* 473–476.

Peterson, C., Villanova, P., & Rapps, C. (1985). Depression and attribution: Factors responsible for inconsistent results in the literature. *Journal of Abnormal Psychology, 94,* 165-168.

Ramsey, R. (1977). Behavioral approaches to bereavement. *Behavior Research and Therapy, 15,* 131-135.

Rando, T. (1984). *Grief, dying, and death: Clinical interventions for caregivers.* Champaign, IL: Research Press.

Rando, T. (1988). *Grieving: How to go on living when someone you love dies.* Lexington, MA: Lexington Books.

Raphael, B. (1983). *The anatomy of bereavement.* New York: Basic Books.

Robinson, P., & Fleming, S. (1989a). Depressotypic cognitive patterns in major depression and conjugal bereavement. Submitted for publication.

Robinson, P., & Fleming, S. (1989b). Differentiating grief and depression. *The Hospice Journal, 5,* 77-88.

Safran, J., Vallis, M., Segal, Z., & Shaw, B. (1986). Assessment of core cognitive processes in cognitive therapy. *Cognitive Therapy and Research, 10,* 509-526.

Schneider, J. (1980, 4th quarter). Clinically significant differences between grief, pathological grief, and depression. *Patient Counselling and Education,* pp. 161-169.

Spitzer, R., & Williams, J. (1984). *Instruction manual for the structured clinical interview for DSM-III (SCID; May 17 revision).* New York: Biometrics Research Department, New York State Psychiatric Institute.

Temes, R. (1980). *Living with an empty chair.* New York: Irvington.

Turco, R. (1981). Regrief treatment facilitated by hypnosis. *American Journal of Hypnosis, 24,* 62-64.

Volkan, V. (1972). The linking objects of pathological mourners. *Archives of General Psychiatry, 27,* 215-221.

Weissman, A., & Beck, A. (1978). *Development and validation of the dysfunctional Attitudes Scale.* Paper presented at the Annual Meeting of the Association for Advancement of Behavior Therapy, Chicago, IL.

Woodfield, R., & Viney, L. (1984-85). A personal construct approach to the conjugally bereaved woman. *Omega: Journal of Death and Dying, 15,* 1-13.

Worden, J. W. (1982). *Grief counseling and grief therapy: A handbook for the mental health practitioner.* New York: Springer.

Wortman, C., & Silver, R. (1989). The myths of coping with loss. *Journal of Consulting and Clinical Psychology, 57,* 349-357.

Zisook, S., & Shuchter, S. (1986). The first four years of widowhood. *Psychiatric Annals, 15,* 288-294.

# 8

# The Application of Cognitive Therapy to Chronic Pain

## Philip C. Miller

## Overview

The purpose of this chapter is to outline the application of cognitive psychotherapy to chronic pain populations. Particular emphasis will be placed on the application of cognitive therapy to patients suffering from musculoskeletal injuries, such as those sustained in motor vehicle or work-related accidents. The nature and prevalence of pain problems will be briefly examined, followed by a consideration of psychological models of the etiology of pain disorders. Cognitive conceptualizations of chronic pain will be discussed, and the clinical implications of these theories will be examined. The following therapeutic issues will be highlighted: (1) the development and maintenance of the therapeutic alliance, (2) flexibility, (3) the role of dysfunctional cognitions in the maintenance of pain disorders, and (4) the importance of considering core cognitions. It will also be argued that cognitive therapy must be undertaken in the context of any psychopathology associated with chronic pain problems. Case examples will be presented to illustrate major points.

## Nature and Prevalence of Chronic Pain Problems

Persistent pain difficulties have been estimated to affect between 11% and 29% of the general population at any given time (Bergened &

---

Philip C. Miller • Behavioral Health Clinic, Toronto, Ontario M6A 2T3, Canada.

Wilson, 1988; Brattberg, Thorslund, & Wikman, 1989; Vonkorff, Dworkin, Laresh, & Cruger, 1988). A recent large-scale American survey of 1,254 individuals, called the Nuprin Study (Sternbach, 1986), estimated that 12.8% of the population suffered from some form of persistent pain difficulty. Although statistics such as these are somewhat difficult to interpret because of the lack of universally accepted defining criteria, these figures do suggest that chronic pain is a common, and therefore significant, problem.

Chronic pain difficulties are generally defined by a persistence of pain for at least six months (Sanders, 1985; Zarkoska & Philips, 1986). This time frame has been accepted by the American Psychiatric Association and is reflected in the DSM-III-R classification of somatoform pain disorder (American Psychiatric Association, 1987). In addition to quantitative factors (e.g., duration), chronic pain is differentiated from acute pain on the basis of qualitative factors. Specifically, chronic pain is associated with affective, behavioral, motivational, and cognitive changes over time (Melzack & Wall, 1982; Sedlack, 1985). As such, there is merit in considering chronic pain as a syndrome in its own right.

Prevalence rates of chronic pain difficulties take on additional significance when considered in light of associated disability. Rates of disability have risen dramatically over the last 30 years, despite estimates that the incidence of pain problems has not significantly changed. Waddell (1987), for example, reports that time lost due to disability increased more than fourfold from 1953 to 1982 in the United Kingdom. Frymoyer *et al.* (1983) estimate that, from 1977 to 1981, the rate of low back pain disability has inreased 14 times the rate of the population growth in the United States.

The costs associated with disability illustrate the enormity of the problem in terms of financial resources. It is estimated that chronic pain difficulties cost upwards of $90 billion annually in the United States (Phillips, 1988). Low back pain alone is estimated to persistently disable approximately 6% of the adult U.S. population (Frymoyer & Catsbaril, 1987), costing in excess of $8 billion annually for medical costs. Canadian statistics are comparable. In Ontario, the Workers' Compensation Board spent over $1.6 billion in compensation benefits in 1988 (Workers' Compensation Board, 1988).

## Conceptualization of Chronic Pain Disorders

A number of models of chronic pain will be presented in this section in order to provide a context for cognitive therapy of pain. The nature of pain is still a matter of speculation, despite its commonality and its survival value as a signal of potential threat to the organism. Theories of pain may be broadly categorized as biomedical, psychological, or bio-psychosocial. *Biomedical* conceptualizations of pain, which focus exclusively on sensory-affective dimensions of the pain experience, have been found to be inadequate to account for the lack of variation between organic pathology and pain response (Liebeskind & Paul, 1977; Weisenberg, 1977).

Melzack and Wall's gate control theory of pain (Melzack & Wall, 1965, 1982) represented a major theoretical development in the field, as it set the stage for broad-based psychological conceptualizations. *Psychological* models of pain are based on a multidimensional perspective, with different models stressing different aspects of the pain experience. For example, behavioral/operant approaches (Fordyce, 1988; Fordyce *et al.*, 1984) focus on the role of observable acts related to pain and illness behavior in maintaining, via differential reinforcement, pain-related disability. Treatment focuses on eliminating dysfunctional pain behaviors and promoting wellness behaviors. Behavioral/respondent approaches (Caldwell & Chase, 1977; Linton, 1985) suggest that pain-related difficulties are maintained by fear associated with movement of painful areas. Fear of pain elicits muscle hypertension, which heightens pain perception and leads to lowered activity levels, with associated physical deconditoning (the pain-fear-atrophy cycle). Treatment approaches focus on physical mobilization, relaxation, and biofeedback.

Cognitive approaches to chronic pain are also characterized by a multidimensional view of pain and related disability (Turk & Flor, 1984). Turk, Meichenbaum, and Genest's (1983) transactional model of pain clearly illustrates the cognitive model. Turk and his colleagues view the pain experience as a dynamic, interpretive process influenced by complex interactions among cognitive/evaluative, emotional/affective, behavioral, and physiological components. Cognitive factors influence the way in which individuals appraise their symptomatology, make decisions regarding health-related and coping behaviors, respond emotionally to their symptoms and disabilities, and utilize the health care system. All these factors, in turn, are viewed as having direct or indirect influences on the subjective phenomenon of pain (i.e., reciprocal determinism; Bandura, 1976). Thus, an individual's belief system, including specific appraisals of ongoing events, previous learning experiences, and attentional processes, all influence pain perception. For example, an individual's emotional and behavioral reaction to a stomach pain interpreted as a symptom of cancer will be much different than that individual's reaction to the same pain interpreted as indigestion from a heavy meal. Interpersonal and familial influences are also regarded as playing a significant role in the development of pain-related attitudes and beliefs (Flor, Turk, & Rudy, 1989; Payne & Norfleet, 1986). Potential targets of intervention derived from this model include coping skills, attitudes concerning self-efficacy and control, maladaptive cognitions pertaining to pain exacerbation, and dysfunctional pain beliefs.

In outlining conceptual models of chronic pain, more general *biopsychosocial* illness behavior models (Engel, 1977; McHugh & Vallis, 1986) should be mentioned. In these models pain is viewed from an even broader perspective, and an attempt is made to integrate biomedical, psychological, and social (including ethnocultural) factors in the conceptualization of illness. Illness behavior models distinguish between disease (physiopathology) and illness (behaviors, attitudes, and symptoms associated with disease which may occur in the absence of disease). The strengths of these models are their comprehensiveness and their emphasis on the equivalence of mediating influences on pain perception without, *a priori*, placing greater emphasis on any one set of factors (see McHugh & Vallis, 1986).

Clearly, there are a number of conceptual models that one could adopt when working with chronic pain patients. Regardless of the model, however, one must deal with the phenomenology of the pain patient. As such, cognitive models are particularly well suited to this population.

## CURRENT COGNITIVE THERAPY APPROACHES WITH CHRONIC PAIN

In this section, a general model of chronic pain, and a treatment model derived from it, will be discussed. This model is largely based on the work of Turk, Meichenbaum, and Genest (1983).

### The Cognitive-Transactional Treatment Model

Cognitive treatment strategies (Corey, 1988; Phillips, 1988; Salkovskis, 1989; Turk *et al.*, 1983) are based on the assumption that chronic pain is exacerbated and perpetuated by maladaptive appraisal and coping. A central principle of treatment is the need to teach patients to reconceptualize their view of their pain. Another central principle is the need to assess and modify coping skills deficits. In order to achieve these goals, Turk *et al.* (1983) have proposed a four-stage treatment model. Their model is particularly useful because it is comprehensive, well articulated, and well grounded in theory. The four stages of treatment are as follows: (1) assessment/reconceptualization/education, (2) skills acquisition, (3) rehearsal and application, and (4) maintenance and follow through.

## Conceptualizaton and Education Stage

Stage 1 involves a detailed assessment, used to develop a case conceptualization, followed by educational activities. Situational analyses, including assessing dimensions of the pain (e.g., severity, temporal pattern), situational determinants, coping styles, life stresses, and social supports, form the bulk of the therapist's initial activities. This assessment often includes obtaining self-report and performance measures as well as interview and collateral reports from significant others.

Educating the patient about a multidimensional view of pain is an essential step toward developing a shared conceptualization of the patient's difficulties. Education is important for a number of reasons. First, it legitimizes the patient's pain experience and suffering. Second, it motivates the patient to mobilize psychological resources in confronting his/her difficulties. Third, it helps the patient to begin the process of reconceptualizing his/her pain difficulties. Fourth, it provides the patient with a framework to guide his/her understanding of the goals, aims, and procedures of the therapy process. Finally, it forms the basis for an active collaborative relationship.

Assessment and reconceptualization of pain problems are intricately intertwined. The very nature of the assessment process (for example, seeking information about situational determinants of pain) implies that pain is multicausal and modifiable. To facilitate reconceptualization, patients' expectations concerning the benefits of therapeutic interventions are elicited. Goal setting, which is introduced in the first stage, also facilitates the reconceptualization of pain as amenable to control and change.

## Skills Acquisition Stage

The skills acquisition stage (stage 2) of Turk *et al.*'s protocol involves teaching specific pain-coping skills and helping the patient accept the value of these skills. Cognitive-behavioral coping strategies include deep muscle relaxation, breathing relaxation, imagery, distraction, reinterpretation of distressing symptoms, activity scheduling, and stress inoculation strategies such as self-instructional training (Meichenbaum, 1985), applied to both pain and other stressful events.

*Rehearsal and Application Stage*

The rehearsal and application stage (stage 3) of treatment involves implementing behavioral techniques (e.g., exercise and physical activities, medication reduction), evaluating social supports, and rehearsal of acquired skills through role playing, imaginal rehearsal, and graded exposure. Irrespective of which techniques are chosen, or indeed, of theoretical orientation, treatment of chronic pain necessitates behavioral interventions designed to reduce disability and increase physical conditioning.

*Follow-Up and Relapse Prevention Stage*

The fourth stage of treatment focuses on follow-up and relapse prevention (see Marlatt & Gordon, 1984) by considering ways to integrate, maintain, and generalize adaptive changes and coping skills.

As illustrated by Turk *et al.*'s (1983) protocol, the development of coping skills is a significant component of treatment. Recently, however, there has been some controversy over the extent to which pain problems result from deficits in coping skills. Even Turk and his colleagues (1983) suggest that there is insufficient evidence to indicate that coping skills deficits alone account for the prevalence of chronic pain disorders. For example, patients with low pain thresholds have been shown to have a repertoire of coping skills (Rosenstiel & Keefe, 1983). Furthermore, there is evidence that spontaneously generated coping strategies are more effective than formally taught coping strategies in dealing with aversive pain situations (Avia & Kanfer, 1980; Stone, Demchik-Stone, & Horan, 1977).

In contrast to the skills deficit model, several authors have suggested that dysfunctional cognitions, such as catastrophizing, interfere with previously acquired coping skills, and as such may account for the variance in coping ability (Avia & Kanfer, 1980; Crook, Tunks, Kalaher, & Roberts, 1988; Reesor & Craig, 1988). Pain sufferers, according to this view, may fail to use effective coping strategies because they feel overwhelmed by the situation. There is some evidence to support this view (Spanos, Radtke-Bordrik, Ferguson, & Jones, 1979; Flor & Turk, 1987; Romano, Tumer, Syrjala, & Levy, 1987). This evidence suggests that therapists need to carefully assess a patient's coping skills repetoire at treatment onset, attempt to identify maladaptive cognitions or situations which interfere with effective coping (Gottleib, 1987), and monitor the patient's self-efficacy (Avia & Kanfer, 1980), rather than focus on coping skills training exclusively.

In summary, cognitive approaches are designed to help the patient change his/her understanding and evaluation of the pain problem, and to provide the patient with adaptive pain and stress coping skills to minimize pain-perpetuating cycles. The approach may be fairly directive, structured, and technique-focused, or unstructured and process-focused. Although Turk and his colleagues emphasize cognitive techniques, they recognize that a variety of cognitive, behavioral, affective, and physical interventions may be effective. The cognitive approach is not defined so much by technique, but by the conceptualizaton of the pain problem and the goals of treatment.

## COGNITIVE THERAPY ISSUES

Current cognitive approaches to the treatment of chronic pain patients provide a useful framework for the therapist. In this section, process, content, and structural issues will be discussed, with the objective of elaborating on standard cognitive approaches.

### Cognitive Process Issues: Rapport and Flexibility

#### Rapport

Whether treatment is offered in the context of a highly structured treatment program (e.g., a 10-session group program) or in an unstructured context (e.g., non-time-limited individual psychotherapy), the development of a strong collaborative therapeutic relationship is essential in effecting treatment success (see Chapter 1, this volume). However, there are a number of therapeutic issues, unique to chronic pain patients, which need to be addressed in order to develop and maintain such a relationship.

Typically, in cognitive therapy, the development of a strong treatment alliance is fostered through educational activities, mutual goal setting, and activities designed to test patients' hypotheses and predictions (Beck, Rush, Shaw, & Emery, 1979). In contrast to patients with non-medical problems, patient skepticism regarding psychological treatments must be addressed with chronic pain patients before educational or goal setting activities are attempted. Typically, pain patients view their problems and symptoms in purely physical terms. Their view is often reinforced by the medical system, where psychological factors are not considered unless other interventions fail. Chronic pain patients are often referred to a psychologist only after many medical/physical interventions have been attempted. Patients may view the referral to a psychologist either as a sign of abandonment by the physician or as an implicit criticism of the validity of their difficulties. Consequently, patients may see little value in undergoing treatment which focuses on psychological factors. It should be noted that such skepticism needs to be dealt with throughout the course of therapy, as it tends to be an ongoing issue.

Lack of acknowledgment or validation of a patient's complaints as genuine by medical professionals and significant others is common with chronic pain problems. This is especially true in cases where physical injuries are relatively minor (see Chapter 5, this volume). As a result, the patient often develops an attitude of hostility and suspiciousness toward health professionals, especially mental health professionals. Consequently, acknowledgment of the patient's complaints and suffering is a necessary first step in the establishment of a positive therapeutic relationship. In many ways, the assessment questions (e.g., "Where does it hurt?" "What makes your pain better?" "What makes it worse?" "What do you think is causing it?") convey acceptance of the seriousness of the patient's complaints and facilitate the development of an alliance. Assessment questions also serve the purpose of providing the clinician with useful information about the patient's personal theories or explanatory models of his/her illness (McHugh & Vallis, 1986). Understanding the patient's existing (pretreatment) explanatory model of his/her pain is a necessary prerequisite for the development of a shared conceptual framework in therapy.

Therapeutic alliance must extend beyond the patient-therapist relationship to include significant others in the patient's life (including family and friends). Pain patients are invariably involved with the medical system and are very often involved with a legal or compensation system as well. Good rapport with the patient's medical doctor and specialist(s) is helpful. Close liasons with other health and legal professionals convey to the patient the legitimacy of his/her problems. This also helps the patient define his/her social support network, while providing a sense that his/her pain problems (because they are complex) are being dealt with in a comprehensive manner. Clear communication with associated professionals concerning the nature of therapy is important, so that referrals may be appropriately made, and treatments may be coordinated.

*Flexibility*

A number of intervention techniques are available to the cognitive therapist, and flexbility in the use of these techniques is therefore important. Techniques may be characterized as cognitive (e.g., imagery, self-hypnosis, self-instruction, stress management) or behavioral (e.g., relaxation, biofeedback, pain behavior extinction). Intervention targets and strategies for change are largely a function of case conceptualization, as well as the patient's needs (see Chapter 2, this volume). For example, one patient was loath to use deep-breathing relaxation because she construed it as yoga, which was contrary to her religious beliefs as a Jehovah's Witness. She was, however, quite comfortable using imagery techniques.

Flexibility in the degree of therapy structure and duration of treatment is also required. Once again, requirements are based on the patient's needs, personality characteristics, and chronicity. It is often unreasonable to expect that the pain patient will attain a specified degree of change in a specified time period, as chronic pain problems are long-standing by definiton. The degree of structure of therapy also depends on the patient's expectations, motivation, insight, initiative, and personality characteristics. While some patients may require a highly directive, structured, closely monitored approach, other patients require very little direction and respond to insight-oriented approaches.

## Cognitive Content Issues: Beliefs about Pain

Since cognitive fators play a significant role in the perception of pain (Turk & Rudy, 1986), it is important to assess and modify those beliefs that impact on the pain experience (Kleinman, 1980; McHugh & Vallis, 1986). There have been a number of attempts to classify relevant dimensions in the explanatory models of pain patients. Williams and Thorn (1989) factor analyzed self-report data, and reported that patients' beliefs concerning their pain tended to fall into seven main content areas: (1) beliefs about the cause of pain, (2) beliefs about the mysterious nature of pain, (3) beliefs about whether pain is experienced constantly or intermittently, (4) beliefs about when pain would remit, (5) beliefs about how pain alters lifestyle, (6) beliefs about personal control of pain, and (7) beliefs regarding blame for pain. Turk, Rudy, and Salovey (1986) found four factors: controllability, seriousness, personal responsibility, and changeability.

In implementing cognitive therapy with chronic pain patients, six categories of beliefs, which subsume the work of Williams and Thorn (1989) and Turk et al. (1986), appear to adequately characterize this population. These six categories (etiology, prognosis, vulnerability, control, disability, and responsibility) are not presented as a taxonomy or model, but rather as a guide to aid the clinician in conceptualizing important cognitions for intervention. Consistent with the notion that assessment interventions are focused on the exploraton of the patient's explanatory model, it is also important to bear in mind that idiosyncratic beliefs may have considerable impact on patient functioning. Consequently, any list of relevant beliefs will be incomplete at best. Nonetheless, flexible interventions addressing the following beliefs are recommended.

### Beliefs about Etiology of Pain

Patients' beliefs about the cause of their pain have significant impact on their rehabilitaton efforts and coping styles. For example, the patient who believes that her back pain is caused by "a pinched nerve" may, despite medical advice to the contrary, continue to seek medical opinions to support her desire for surgery to rectify the problem. Williams and Thorn (1989) found that individuals who believed the cause of their pain to be mysterious (without definite cause) tended to have greater difficulty with psychological treatment adherence and reported lower self-esteem. It is not surprising that beliefs about the cause of pain have significant impact on treatment adherence, as they are highly associated with the credibility of various treatment modalities. Patients often have fairly clearly defined notions concerning the sorts of treatment modalities which will help them. For example, a patient with low back pain, who had experienced relief by a previous discotomy, believed that the next-higher disc was causing the problem and wanted further surgery to remove it.

It is important to note that patients are often reluctant to share their beliefs about causality when asked by the clinician, for fear of intruding into the professional's domain. By asking patients what understanding of their pain problems they have received from their doctors (e.g., "What have your doctors told you is the cause of your pain?"), the clinician may desensitize patients to a discussion of their own beliefs. Providing structure in the form of querying specific locations of their pain (e.g., "Do you believe it's in your muscles, nerves, bones?") or citing common fears (e.g., "Do you think the headaches are a sign of a brain tumor or cancer?") often facilitates an assessment of etiological beliefs.

The content of causal beliefs can vary from vague or nonexistent to bizarre. Undifferentiated beliefs about cause ("I don't know the cause," "I'm not a doctor," "I just want to get better") combined with an attitude of overreliance on medical practitioners ("I just do what my doctor tells me") may be a sign of passivity and poor motivation for treatment. If the patient-physician relationship is a strong one, enlisting the support of the physician to encourage more active approaches may be useful.

In addition to the content differences in causal beliefs, the amenability of these beliefs to corrective feedback, consideration of alternatives, testing out beliefs, or hypothesis testing is an essential clinical issue. In many cases, erroneous beliefs are based on lack of information or misinformation about cause and, as such, are readily correctable by simply providing information. For example, providing information concerning the failure rate of discotomies and the symptoms associated with lumbar disc disease may be sufficient to help the previously mentioned patient accept the treatment failure.

Not all dysfunctional causal beliefs are amenable to education/feedback, however. Other treatment approaches to develop more adaptive causal beliefs are available to the clinician. Encouraging the patient to test predictions based on the causal beliefs and, in doing so, reappraise them may be effective. For example, pain patients commonly anticipate dire consequences (e.g., having a heart attack, breaking a disc fusion, having a stroke) of engaging in exercise after prolonged periods of inactivity. Symptoms of deconditioning (fatigue, chest pain, dizziness, shortness of breath) are often misinterpreted as symptoms of illness. Helping patients confront these fears necessitates graded exposure to feared activities.

In other cases, it may be necessary to explore the personal meaning associated with beliefs of causality. For example, in the case of the previously cited low back pain patient, the issue of the personal meaning of failed surgery had much more clinical significance than her beliefs of pain etiology. By exploring the meaning of failure with the patient, she could come to terms with the fact that surgery had not, in her case, been successful. This, in turn, opened up avenues for coping with her pain problem rather than searching for an unrealistic cure.

With a chronic pain population, the credibility of the information-giver may be a salient issue. Patients do not always credit the authority of a nonmedical practitioner when information is of a highly technical or medical nature. Rereferral to a medical practitioner (one whom the patient trusts or holds in high regard) specifically for the purpose of education concerning cause may be necessary.

## Beliefs about Course and Prognosis

Beliefs about prognosis of pain also have a significant impact on coping ability, treatment adherence, and pain perception. Williams and Thorn (1989) found that beliefs that pain was enduring were associated with lower treatment adherence and self-esteem, and increased self-reported pain intensity. Interestingly, beliefs about unrelenting pain were unrelated to actual pain duration in their sample, suggesting that factors other than actual chronicity influence beliefs about prognosis.

Of particular importance for the clinician is the impact of beliefs about prognosis on motivation for, and adherence to, treatment. These beliefs might be considered as analogous in some ways to the negative view of the future component of the negative cognitive triad in depression (Beck *et al.*, 1979). In fact, many of the techniques used to combat hopelessness with a depressed population (Beck *et al.*, 1979), such as challenging the logic of pessimistic predictions, and encouraging behaviors incompatible with the predicted outcome (with pain patients these are pain incompatible behaviors), can be applied directly to a chronic pain population.

Beliefs about etiology and prognosis are often highly interrelated, as the patient's outlook depends largely on his/her notions of cause. Consequently, those techniques or approaches which influence causal beliefs may indirectly influence prognostic beliefs as well. Specifically, self-instructional training, analysis of the grounds for pessimism, exploration of the advantages and disadvantages of prognostic beliefs, and analysis of negative behavioral and emotional consequences of pessimistic beliefs may be used in these situations.

Another approach to challenging beliefs about prognosis is to encourage suspended judgment about the future ("let's wait and see"). If this is possible, patients may be more willing to commit themselves to cognitive therapy. Beliefs about prognosis often change in response to progress in therapy, with patients becoming more optimistic as they increase daily functioning and increase their sense of personal effectiveness. Consequently, periodic reevaluation of beliefs concerning prognosis throughout the course of therapy is recommended.

## Beliefs concerning Vulnerability to Reinjury

It is not uncommon for chronic pain patients to develop the belief that they are highly vulnerable to reinjury or further damage from engaging in specific physical activities. Such beliefs can mediate avoidance of activity (Fordyce *et al.*, 1981). For example, low back pain patients commonly believe that activities which aggravate back pain, such as bending or lifting, will cause further damage to their back (e.g., will cause paralysis or will cause a disc to slip). The resultant inactive lifestyle can perpetuate pain difficulties in a variety of ways, such as through the risk of muscle atrophy, depression, lessened sense of control, and loss of self-esteem. This dynamic may, in part, explain the relationship between chronic pain and lowered self-esteem observed in depressed pain patients by Kerns and Turk (1984).

Assessment of beliefs in vulnerability to reinjury involves evaluating the damage or injury that patients believe pain-related activites will result in. Questions such as the following are useful here: "When pain is intense, what do you think is going on?" "What damage do you think will happen if you do such and such?" and "What activities have your doctors told you to avoid?" Cognitions concerning damage are not always readily assessable in interview situations because of their possible situational specificity. It may be necessary to have patients monitor automatic thoughts in pain-producing situations. Exposing patients to pain-producing activities *in vivo* is a powerful way to access maladaptive cognitions. The success of home-based outpatient pain management programs (e.g., Corey, Etlin, & Miller, 1987) may in some ways be accounted for by the *in vivo* assessment and treatment opportunities.

It is also important to assess both immediate and retrospective appraisals of the initial trauma in the case of accident victims. Questions such as the following are useful here: "When you were injured, what did you think happened to you?" "What did your doctors tell you then?" and "Looking back on the situation, what injuries did you sustain?" Often lack of information, or misinformation, concerning the nature of injuries sustained contributes to beliefs in vulnerability. The extent to which the initial trauma contributes to a generalized sense of vulnerability is a question which deserves further research. Clinical experience indicates that fears of reinjury and a sense of victimization may generalize to new situations, as occurs with posttraumatic stress disorder patients (see Chapter 5, this volume).

Drawing a distinction between "hurt" (discomfort) and "harm" (damage) is often an initial step in the process of helping patients reappraise the risk of engaging in pain-producing physical activities (Cott, 1986). Patients should be encouraged to avoid only activities that harm, not activities that hurt. This may take place in the form of a general discussion about the nature of pain, or a discussion of pain "myths" (Miller, 1986). Further, encouraging patients to encounter feared situations in a graded manner is necessary to effect reevaluation and induce more adaptive appraisals. Imaginal exposure is, in the author's experience, largely ineffective. Furthermore, when designing an exposure hierarchy, it is recommended that hierarchical tasks simulate as closely as possible the desired goal task, as generalization from a simulated task may be low. For example, if a patient would like to take out his garbage but is afraid of lifting and bending, it is more effective to set up a behavioral schedule involving lifting garbage cans of increasing weight rather than to set up a schedule involving bending and lifting weights in a gym.

*Beliefs concerning Personal Control of Pain*

The perception of personal control over stressful life events has been shown to be a significant stress modifier with a number of clinical populations (Lefcourt, 1982; Silver & Wortman, 1980), including pain populations (Crisson & Keefe, 1988). One of the most significant cognitive factors in the development of pain-associated depression may be beliefs concerning lack of control over pain and associated symptoms (Bowers, 1968). Seligman's (1975) learned helplessness model of depression has particular relevance for pain patients. If patients have little control over pain or associated emotional symptoms, they may develop a generalized helplessness response to chronic, aversive, uncontrollable pain stimuli. This is often seen in clinical practice when patients, as a result of loss of self-efficacy due to unsuccessful attempts to cope with pain, lose confidence in areas of their life unaffected by pain. For example, a formerly assertive salesman was unable to request that a fellow bus passenger desist from smoking in a nonsmoking area. In turn, development of a helplessness response to pain and other life events may further undermine successful coping, in a cyclic pattern.

Recognizing the importance of personal control of symptoms, cognitive-behavioral treatment programs tend to utilize a variety of techniques (e.g., muscle relaxation, imagery, distraction, and coping self-statements) to help patients modify pain symptoms and associated emotional reactions (Gottlieb, 1987). Recent research is beginning to examine the relative efficacy of these techniques as they impact on views of personal control (Fernandez & Turk, 1989).

Treatment interventions that focus on the management of stressful life events are based on assumptions that life stresses can exacerbate pain and a generalized loss of effectiveness can result from ineffective attempts to control pain. Consequently, stress management skills including assertiveness are commonly reviewed with patients. The impact of successful stress management is reviewed with respect to the patient's overall sense of self-efficacy.

*Beliefs concerning Disability*

The disability caused by chronic pain is, understandably, a major area of concern for patients, family, and the health care system. However, there is some evidence to suggest that chronic pain patients are inaccurate in their perception of disability (Fordyce *et al.*, 1984). Gallon (1989), for example, found that in long-term follow-up of a multidisciplinary low back treatment program, successful (less disabled) candidates still perceived themselves as disabled, despite their high func-

tioning on objective measures of vocational status, compensation benefits, and medication use. In contrast, unsuccessful (more disabled) candidates were more accurate in their perception of disability. These results suggest that, consistent with clinial observation, pain patients may
underestimate their physical abilities (Linton, 1985). Misconceptions of
disability tend to undermine successful coping, may have a negative
impact on self-efficacy judgments, and may contribute to failure to
maintain treatment gains. In fact, one possible reason for the high relapse rate in many pain management programs (Malec, Cayner, Harvey,
& Timming, 1981; Maruta, Swanson, & McHardy, 1987) is the possible
failure to modify patients' beliefs in personal ineffectiveness and helplessness, despite increases in functioning.

Gallon's (1989) results suggest the importance of targeting patients'
cognitions of disability as well as their actual functioning level. Monitoring and providing accurate feedback of functioning ability helps to
clarify the individual's perception of his/her functioning and may assist
in modifying beliefs of disability. Behavioral interventions, such as
graded exposure and exercise, target disability behavior directly, and as
such may challenge beliefs of disability as well as behavioral avoidance.
Techniques to enhance ability to cope with life stressors (such as stress
inoculation training, problem solving, coping self-statements) also enhance self-efficacy, which in turn contributes to increased emotional and
physical functioning. For example, patients need to focus on areas of
successful coping rather than dwell on those areas of disability and
unsuccessful coping. Chronic pain patients often undermine successful
coping by dwelling on areas of functioning which continue to be difficult
("I know I can walk 10 minutes now, but I still can't work even part-
time").

### Beliefs about Personal Responsibility for Pain

Patients frequently voice the concern that their pain problems are
much more difficult to cope with as a result of being caused by the
carelessness or, in some cases, the intention of others. These external
attributions and associated feelings can have particular impact during
severe pain or stress episodes, when aversive stimuli trigger thoughts of
blame and feelings of helplessness and anger. For example, an airline
attendant with neck pain resulting from a personal assault incurred
when he was protecting a passenger developed rage responses to increases in pain and also developed ongoing homicidal ideation.

Blaming others for pain difficulties is often an issue for postaccident, postassault or, in some cases, postoperative pain patients, and is
often associated with feelings of victimization. These patients often be-

lieve that their pain difficulties would be easier to cope with if they were self-inflicted, because they would feel less angry and less a victim of someone else's negligence.

Negative self-appraisal, in the form of self-recrimination, is also commonly found in the chronic pain population. In the case of accident victims, patients may blame themselves for the accident that caused their pain difficulties. Negative self-appraisals may be part of a more generalized negative cognitive set characteristic of depression and loss of confidence which often accompanies unsuccessful coping (Calhoun, Chency, & Dawes, 1974).

A particular type of self-blame that needs to be assessed in the case of survivors of accidents that result in fatalities involves survivor guilt. Self-blame may also result from characterological assumptions which may manifest in the form of self-recriminations concerning lack of treatment progress ("I'm no good," "No treatment will help someone like me.") In such cases, the meaning of treatment progress vis-à-vis the self needs to be explored. Often, accidents call into question patients' views of justice and their belief in a just world (Lerner, 1980). Assessing the consequences associated with justice, retribution, and concern by the third party is valuable in determining the extent to which patients have resolved issues of blame. For example, one might ask whether the third party was charged and whether any criminal action was taken for negligence. One might be interested in finding out the outcome of criminal action or whether the third party displayed any signs of remorse toward the victim.

Since both external attributions ("It's his fault, the idiot") and negative internal attributions about the cause of pain problems can undermine successful coping, therapeutic interventions should focus on helping patients make the appropriate cognitive shifts. Where patients have conflicts concerning unresolved anger toward a third party, efforts are made to work through that anger. Impulse control strategies (Novaco, 1975) are effective not only in helping patients control anger, but also in reappraising aversive situations from the external ("The injury wrecked my life") to the internal ("How can I handle this situation?"). Where patients demonstrate negative self-appraisals ("I deserve to be in pain right now for killing that woman"), therapeutic interventions are focused on shifting attributions from dysfunctional to adaptive.

## Cognitive Structural Issues: Changing Core Beliefs

So far, interventions directed at the level of cognitive content have been discussed. However, interventions at the level of core cognitive structures are sometimes needed to effect change. As discussed in Chapter 2 (this volume), cognitions may be viewed as occurring at a variety of levels (e.g., peripheral and core levels). Cognitive dysfunctions may occur at any level of the hierarchy. From this perspective, interventions are assumed to be most effective when matched with the level of cognitive dysfunction. That is, if a patient's chronic pain problems are conceptualized as resulting from dysfunctions at the level of cognitive structures or core cognitive constructs ("I am unlovable and I deserve to live in pain"), interventions at this level are most likely to result in lasting change. An examination of core cognitive processes, therefore, may be warranted when standard cognitive therapy interventions (Beck *et al.*, 1979; Turk *et al.*, 1983) fail, since core beliefs and attitudes may interfere with adaptive coping. For example, it is not uncommon, when treating accident victims, to find premorbid coping styles based on core beliefs about the self which are no longer adaptive. As discussed in Chapter 2 (this volume), it may be necessary to go beyond an examination of content-level issues and explore beliefs at the level of cognitive process or structure in order to effect change. Also, attempting to modify dysfunctional core beliefs may promote changes at the level of cognitive content, which would facilitate pain coping. Consider the following case example as an illustration of this point.

> Mr. C., a baker in his 20s, suffering from neck and low back pain following a work-related injury, was referred by a colleague because he had difficulty complying with a behavioral strategy designed to regulate his activity level. He had developed a pattern of intense overactivity for a number of days followed by prolonged inactivity, a pattern typical of chronic pain patients. He was only able to work part-time postaccident and had developed impulse control problems and rage responses which were causing severe family distress.
>
> Personal history revealed that Mr. C. had had learning difficulties as a child, which not only had disrupted his schooling and caused him to have difficulty forming social relationships, but had also incurred the disapproval of his father, whom Mr. C. greatly admired. In order to deal with these difficulties, Mr. C. had elected at a fairly early age to become a baker, a vocation at which he could excel by reasons of perseverance and hard work. He had worked as a baker since his early teens. He customarily worked 60 to 70 hours per week preaccident, often working overtime without pay. As well, his diligent work record had gained him the approval and respect of his father.
>
> Over a period of a number of sessions, the following conceptualization of important core beliefs for Mr. C. was developed. In many ways, he functioned in a manner in which approval was only available through high achievement in his career. As well, he was highly competitive, believing

that in order to achieve, he must be more productive than his competitors. In fact, Mr. C. stated "the only way to be worthwhile is to be the best baker there is." This had resulted in a compulsive coping style, a style which contributed to his postaccident adjustment difficulties. For example, he found it very difficult to pace his activities, since he believed that he had to get tasks finished without interruption or breaks. It was further hypothesized that inability to meet his internalized productivity expectations postaccident led to aggressive reactions, as a result of frustration.

Throughout the course of these sessions, the behavioral strategy of scheduling activities was reintroduced in the context of exploring these fundamental beliefs concerning worth. As Mr. C. was able to to reappraise his internal standards of self-respect, he was also able to reappraise the value of scheduling his activity as a pain-coping skill. Consequently, he was able to draw up a daily timetable and follow that timetable. He was more able to limit his activities, according to that timetable, rather than pushing himself to the point where he experienced significant pain increases.

This example illustrates the need to examine core belief issues in cases where content-based attempts to change coping style fail. It is quite likely that failure to address core concerns in this case would have led to Mr. C. continuing to use a compulsive coping style, failing to respond to efforts to structure his activities, and consequently, being unable to reduce pain or increase functioning. Thus, direct examination of the underlying issues contributing to his maladaptive coping facilitated therapeutic change.

## PSYCHOPATHOLOGY ASSOCIATED WITH CHRONIC PAIN DISORDERS

There is reliable evidence of associations between chronic pain and depression (Atkinson, Slater, Grant, Patterson, & Garfin, 1988; Romano & Turner, 1985), anxiety (Marlow, West, & Sutkin, 1989), stress (Feuerstein, Carter, & Papciak, 1987), and marital and sexual difficulties (Flor, Turk, & Rudy, 1989; Hafstrom & Schram, 1984; Infante, 1981). In the case of accident victims, posttraumatic stress disorder may also occur (see Chapter 5, this volume). Consequently, case conceptualization and interventon is largely dictated by the particular constellation of symptoms and emotional difficulties with which the clinician is confronted. In some cases, emotional difficulties may be masked or overlooked, especially if patients are preoccupied with pain complaints. Associated life stresses, premorbid issues, and developmental issues, also compound the presentation.

Typically, cognitive therapy with chronic pain patients progresses from an initial focus on pain-related problems to a discussion of personal and related issues. However, pain problems remain of primary concern to chronic pain patients whether or not they are the immediate focus of therapy at any particular point in time. Contrary to a psychoanalytic perspective (Blumer & Heilbronn, 1982), pain problems are not viewed as a manifestation of deeper issues, but are viewed as problems in their own right. The following case example illustrates this perspective, and the importance of dealing with related personal problems in therapy.

Mr. D., a stockbroker in his 40s, presented with pain in the right leg and foot following fractures sustained in a motor vehicle accident. He had developed anxiety symptoms of a generalized nature postaccident. He attempted to deal with these by excessive ingestion of alcohol to the point where he was concerned about alcohol abuse. Tragically, his father committed suicide three months postaccident. He partially blamed himself for his father's death because of his own prolonged disability. He felt that his disability was a source of stress to his father, which contributed to his taking his own life.

A number of sessions were spent working through Mr. D.'s grief. He had received medical treatment for over two years but had not had any opportunity to discuss his concerns about his father's loss. Mr. D. also raised issues concerning the care of his teenage child (he was a single parent). He had questions about goals and values when his son reached adulthood and left home. By discussing these issues, reappraising them, and putting them in perspective (he was not responsible for his father's death), he made improvements in other areas of his life without these areas being specific targets of therapy. At this point in therapy, Mr. D. remarked that he was feeling better emotionally, was no longer having anxiety difficulties, had stopped drinking, and had begun to socialize, something which he had not done for many years. He had never had an intimate relationship since separation from his wife many years prior to the accident.

After having made these gains, Mr. D. reintroduced concerns about his pain problems. At that point, full attention was paid to the pain problems, with recommendations concerning coping and alleviation. Relaxation procedures were taught, imagery techniques were implemented, and Mr. D. learned to use self-instructional strategies to cope with periods of severe pain. Over time, connections were made between pain difficulties and the issues pertaining to loss (e.g., unresolved grief was a stressor contributing to aggravation of pain).

This case example illustrates a number of points. First, emotional disturbance associated with pain difficulties merits appropriate assessment and intervention. Second, pain problems remain a focus of concern and a target of intervention irrespective of related issues. Third, flexibility in terms of the timing of interventions is very important. If Mr. D. had been offered a more structured, symptom-focused pain management approach without first having an opportunity to explore emotional concerns, pain difficulties may have been focused on to the exclusion of his concerns of unresolved grief, and therapy may have failed.

## CONCLUSIONS

The purpose of this chapter was to offer treatment guidelines to the cognitive therapist working with chronic pain patients. Current psychological models of chronic pain and standard content-based cognitive therapy approaches were reviewed. A number of therapeutic issues were then discussed. At the level of cognitive process and content, issues pertaining to rapport, flexibility, and beliefs about pain were considered. At the level of cognitive structure, issues pertaining to core beliefs and their impact on pain coping were considered. Finally, pain problems were discussed in the context of associated psychopathology.

There is increasing evidence that cognitive therapy is effective in the treatment of chronic pain difficulties (Anderson, Cole, Gullickson, Hudgens, & Roberts, 1977; Corey et al., 1987; Guck, Skultety, Meilman, & Dowd, 1985). At the present time, the primary treatment research questions pertain to discovering the most efficient and powerful applications of cognitive therapy, and to identifying significant mechanisms of change. More information is required concerning what aspects of the therapeutic process are instrumental in affecting change, and what approaches are most effective with different personality styles. Further research is needed to address how generalizable treatment findings are across pain populations, since chronic pain patients represent an extremely heterogenous group.

Another major research issue pertains to early intervention and prevention of disability. Preliminary data collected from a sample of injured workers at our clinic (the Behavioral Health Clinic, Toronto) suggest that intervention earlier than one year postaccident is more effective than intervention later than one year. Using termination of compensation benefit status as the criterion of success, 46% of the sample treated within one year of injury were successful, while only 29% of the sample treated later than one year postinjury were successful. This is consistent with findings that indicate that positive prognosis and rehabilitation potential decreases with time since symptom onset (White, 1969).

There have been a number of important theoretical developments in cognitive therapy (see Chapter 1, this volume) which, as discussed in this text, may have tremendous treatment implications. Further development of these perspectives, and investigation of their applicability to the treatment of chronic pain patients, holds promise for the future. However, in Ontario, Canada, at least, there is increasing economic and political pressure to provide pain management services with greater cost effectiveness. This pressure may lead to increasingly structured programs and may act as a retarding force to the diversifying trends in theoretical development and clinical application.

In summary, there is a clear need to integrate theoretical developments and clinical application. At the same time, there is a need to validate proposed intervention strategies. To echo Turk, Meichenbaum, and Genest's (1983) caution, there is tremendous potential for harm if unvalidated treatment approaches are implemented, even if they are theoretically sound.

ACKNOWLEGMENTS. I would like to acknowledge the assistance of Dr. Louise Koepfler in the preparation of this chapter. I would also like to acknowledge the support of my wife, Linda, and son, Christopher, during its preparation.

# REFERENCES

American Psychiatric Association (1987). *Diagnostic and statistical manual of mental disorders* (3rd edition, revised). Washington, DC: Author.

Anderson, T. P., Cole, T. M., Gullickson, G., Hudgens, A., & Roberts, A. H. (1977). Behavior modification of chronic pain. A treatment program by a multidisciplinary team. *Clinical Orthopaedics and Related Research, 129,* 96-100.

Atkinson, J. H., Slater, M. A., Grant, I., Patterson, T. L., & Garfin, S. R. (1988). Depressed mood in chronic low back pain: Relationship with stressful life events. *Pain, 35,* 47-56.

Avia, M. D., & Kanfer, F. H. (1980). Coping with aversive stimulation: The effects of training in a self-management context. *Cognitive Therapy and Research, 4,* 73-81.

Bandura, A. (1976). *Social learning theory.* Englewood Cliffs, NJ: Prentice Hall.

Beck, A. T., Rush, A. J., Shaw, B., & Emery, G. (1979). *Cognitive therapy of depression.* New York: Guilford.

Bergened, H., & Wilson, B. (1988). Back pain in middle age: Occupational workload and psychologic factors: An epidemiological survey. *Spine, 13,* 58-60.

Blumer, D., & Heilbronn, M. (1982). Chronic pain as a variant of depressive disease. The pain-prone disorder. *Journal of Nervous and Mental Disease, 170,* 381-406.

Bowers, K. S. (1968). Pain, anxiety, and perceived control. *Journal of Consulting and Clinical Psychology, 32,* 596-602.

Brattberg, G., Thorslund, M., & Wikman, A. (1989). The prevalence of pain in a general population. The results of a postal survey in a county of Sweden. *Pain, 37*(2), 215-222.

Caldwell, A. B., & Chase, C. (1977). Diagnosis and treatment of personality factors in chronic low back pain. *Clinical Orthopaedics and Related Research, 129,* 141-149.

Calhoun, L. G., Chency, T., & Dawes, A. S. (1974). Locus of control, self-reported depression, and perceived causes of depression. *Journal of Consulting and Clinical Psychology*, 42, 736.

Corey, D. (1988). *Pain: Learning to live without it*. Toronto: McMillan.

Corey, D. T., Etlin, D., & Miller, P. C. (1987). A home-based pain management and rehabilitation programme: An evaluation. *Pain*, 29, 219-229.

Cott, A. (1986). The disease-illness distinction: A model for effective and practical integration of behavioral and medical sciences. In S. McHugh & T. M. Vallis (Eds.), *Illness behavior: A multidisciplinary model* (pp. 72-100). New York: Plenum.

Crisson, J. E., & Keefe, F. J. (1988). The relationship of locus of control to pain coping strategies and psychological distress in chronic pain patients. *Pain*, 35(2), 147-154.

Crook, J., Tunks, E., Kalaher, S., & Roberts, J. (1988). Coping with persistent pain: A comparison of persistent pain sufferers in a specialty clinic and in a family practice clinic. *Pain*, 34, 175-184.

Engel, G. (1977). The need for a new medical model: A challenge for biomedicine. *Science*, 196, 129-136.

Fernandez, E., & Turk, D. C. (1989). The utility of cognitive coping strategies for altering pain perception: A meta-analysis. *Pain*, 38, 123-136.

Feuerstein, M., Carter, R. L., & Papciak, A. S. (1987). A prospective analysis of stress and fatigue in recurrent low back pain. *Pain*, 31, 333-344.

Flor, H., & Turk, D. C. (1987). *Pain-related cognitions, pain severity, and pain behaviors in chronic pain patients*. Paper Presented to the Fifth World Congress on Pain, International Association for the Study of Pain, Hamburg, FRG.

Flor, H., Turk, D. C., & Rudy, T. E. (1989). Relationship of pain impact and significant other reinforcement of pain behaviors: The mediating role of gender, marital status and marital satisfaction. *Pain*, 38, 35-44.

Fordyce, W. E. (1988). The behavioral management of pain, a critique of a critique. *Pain*, 33, 35-387.

Fordyce, W. E., McMahon, R., Rainwater, G., Jackins, S., Questad,K., Murphy, T., & Delateur, B. (1981). Pain complaint exercise performance relationship in chronic pain. *Pain*, 10, 311-321.

Fordyce, W. E., Lansky, D., Calsyn, D. A., Sheltn, J. L., Stolov, W. C., & Lock, D. S. (1984). Pain measurement and pain behavior. *Pain*, 18, 53-69.

Frymoyer, J. W., & Catsbaril, W. (1987). Predictors of low back pain disability. *Clinical Orthopaedics and Related Research*, 221, 89-98.

Frymoyer, J. W., Pope, M. H., Clements, J., Wilder, D., MacPherson, B., & Ashkaga, T. (1983). Risk factors in low-back pain. *Journal of Bone and Joint Surgery*, 65a, 213-216.

Gallon, R. L. (1989). Perception of disability in chronic back pain patients: A long-term follow-up. *Pain*, 37(1), 67-76.

Gottlieb, B. S. (1987). *A cognitive therapy approach to chronic pain*. Paper presented to the Fifth World Congress on Pain, International Association for the Study of Pain, Hamburg, FRG.

Guck, T. P., Skultety, F. M., Meilman, P. W., & Dowd, E. T. (1985). Multidisciplinary pain center follow-up study: Evaluation with a no-treatment control group. *Pain*, 21, 295-306.

Hafstrom, J. L., & Schram, V. R. (1984). Chronic illness in couples: Selected characteristics, including wives' satisfaction with and perception of marital relationships. *Family Relations*, 33, 195-203.

Infante, M. C. (1981). Sexual dysfunction in the patient with chronic back pain. *Sexual Disability*, 4, 173-178.

Kerns, R. D., & Turk, D. C. (1984). Depression and chronic pain: The mediating role of the spouse. *Journal of Marriage and the Family, 46*, 845-852.

Kleinman, A. (1980). *Patients and healers in the context of culture*. Berkeley: University of California Press.

Lefcourt, H. M. (1982). *Locus of control: Current trends in theory and research* (2nd edition). HIllsdale, NJ: Erlbaum.

Lerner, M. J. (1980). *The belief in a just world*. New York: Plenum.

Liebeskind, J. C., & Paul, L. A. (1977). Psychological and physiological mechanisms of pain. *Annual Review of Psychology, 28*, 41-60.

Linton, S. J. (1985). The relationship between activity and chronic back pain. *Pain, 21*, 289-294.

Malec, J., Cayner, J. J., Harvey, R. K., & Timming, R. C. (1981). Pain management: Long-term follow-up of an in-patient program. *Archives of Physical Medicine and Rehabilitation, 62*, 369-372.

Marlatt, A., & Gordon, J. (1984). *Relapse prevention: A self-control strategy for the maintenance of behavior change*. New York: Guilford.

Marlow, R., West, J., & Sutkin, P. (1989). Anxiety and pain response changes across treatment: Sensory decision analysis. *Pain, 38*, 35-44.

Maruta, T., Swanson, D. W., & McHardy, M. J. (1987). *Three-year follow-up of patients with chronic pain who were treated in a multidisciplinary pain management program*. Paper presented to the Fifth World Congress on Pain, International Association for the Study of Pain, Hamburg, FRG.

McHugh, S., & Vallis, T. M. (1986). Illness behavior: Operationalization of the bio-psychosocial model. In S. McHugh & T. M. Vallis (Eds.), *Illness behavior: A multi-disciplinary model* (pp. 1-32). New York: Plenum.

Miller, R. S. (1986). Psychological approaches to chronic pain: Assessment and treatment. *The Advocate's Quarterly, 17*(2), 148-155.

Meichenbaum, D. (1985). *Stress inoculation training*. New York: Pergamon Press.

Melzack, R., & Wall, P. (1965). Pain mechanisms: A new theory. *Science, 50*, 971-979.

Melzack, R., & Wall, P. (1982). *The challenge of pain* (rev. edition). London: Penguin Books.

Novaco, R. W. (1975). *Anger control: The development and evaluation of an experimental treatment*. Lexington, MA: Lexington Books.

Payne, B., & Norfleet, M. A. (1986). Chronic pain and the family: A review. *Pain, 26*, 1-22.

Phillips, H. C. (1988). *The psychological management of chronic pain: A treatment manual*. New York: Springer.

Reesor, K. A., & Craig, K. D. (1988). Medically incongruent chronic back pain: Physical limitations, suffering and inefficient coping. *Pain, 32*, 35-45.

Romano, J. M., & Turner, J. A. (1985). Chronic pain and depression: Does the evidence support a relationship. *Psychological Bulletin, 97*, 18-34.

Romano, J. M., Turner, J. A., Syrjala, K. L., & Levy, R. L. (1987). *Coping strategies of chronic pain patients: Relationship to patient characteristics and functioning*. Paper presented to the Fifth World Congress on Pain, International Association for the Study of Pain, Hamburg, FRG.

Rosenstiel, A. K., & Keefe, F. J. (1983). The use of cognitive coping strategies in chronic low back pain patients: Relationship to patient characteristics and current adjustment. *Pain, 17*, 33-44.

Salkovskis, P. (1989). Somatic problems. In P. Hawton, P. Salkovskis, J. Kirk, & D. Clark (Eds.), *Cognitive behavior therapy for psychiatric problems* (pp. 235-276). New York: Oxford University Press.

Sanders, S. H. (1985). Chronic pain: Conceptualization and epidemiology. *Annals Behavioral Medicine, 7*, 3-5.

Sedlack, K. (1985). Low back pain. Perception and tolerance. *Spine, 10*, 440-444.

Seligman, M. E. (1975). *Helplessness: On depression, development and death.* San Francisco: W. H. Freeman.

Silver, R. L., & Wortman, C. B. (1980). Coping with undesirable life events. In J. Garber & M. E. Seligman (Eds.), *Human helplessness.* New York: Academic Press.

Spanos, N. P., Radtke-Bordrik, H. L., Ferguson, J. D., & Jones, B. (1979). The effects of hypnotic susceptibility, suggestions for analgesia, and the utilization of cognitive strategies on the reduction of pain. *Journal of Abnormal Psychology, 88*, 282-292.

Steinbach, R. A. (1986). Survey of pain in the United States: The Nuprin pain report. *Clinical Journal of Pain, 2*, 49-54.

Stone, C. I., Demchik-Stone, D. A., & Horan, J. J. (1977). Coping with pain: A component analysis of Lamaze and cognitive-behavioral procedures. *Journal of Psychosomatic Research, 21*, 451-456.

Turk, D. C., & Flor, H. (1984). Etiological theories and treatments for chronic back pain. II. Psychological models and interventions. *Pain, 19*, 209-233.

Turk, D., & Rudy, T. E. (1986). Assessment of cognitive factors in chronic pain: A worthwhile enterprise? *Journal of Consulting and Clinical Psychology, 54*, 760-768.

Turk, D. C., Meichenbaum, D., & Genest, M. (1983). *Pain and behavioral medicine: A cognitive-behavioral perspective.* New York: Guilford.

Turk, D., Rudy, T., & Salovey, P. (1986). Implicit models of illness. *Journal of Behavioral Medicine, 9*, 453-474.

VonKorff, M., Dworkin, S. F., Laresh, L., & Kruger, A. (1988). An epidemiological comparison of pain complaints. *Pain, 32*, 173-183.

Waddell, G. (1987). A new clinical model for the treatment of low-back pain. *Spine, 12*, 632-644.

Weisenburg, M. (1977). Pain and pain control. *Psychological Bulletin, 84*, 1008-1044.

White, A. W. M. (1969). Low back pain in men receiving workmen's compensation: A follow-up study. *Canadian Medical Association Journal, 101*, 61-67.

Williams, D. A., & Thorn, B. E. (1989). An empirical assessment of pain beliefs. *Pain, 36* (3), 351.

Workers' Compensation Board of Ontario. (1988). *Annual report 1988.* Research and Publications Dept., Workers' Compensation Board of Ontario.

Zarkowska, E., & Philips, H. C. (1986). Recent onset vs. persistent pain: Evidence for a distinction. *Pain, 25*, 365-372.

# Index